THE
LOTTE BERK
METHOD
OF EXERCISE

THE LOTTE BERK METHOD OF EXERCISE

Lotte Berk & Jean Prince

Designed by Mike Jarvis
Text photography by Bob Marchant

QUARTET BOOKS
LONDON MELBOURNE NEW YORK

To all my faithful students, and to
my loyal assistant Lois Complin,
who so beautifully modelled the
exercises in this book.

LOTTE BERK

First published by Quartet Books Limited 1978
A member of the Namara Group
27 Goodge Street, London W1P 1FD

Text copyright © 1978 by Jean Prince
Photographs copyright © 1978 by Quartet Books Limited

ISBN 0 7043 3218 3

Printed in Great Britain by
Hazell Watson & Viney Ltd, Aylesbury, Bucks

Contents

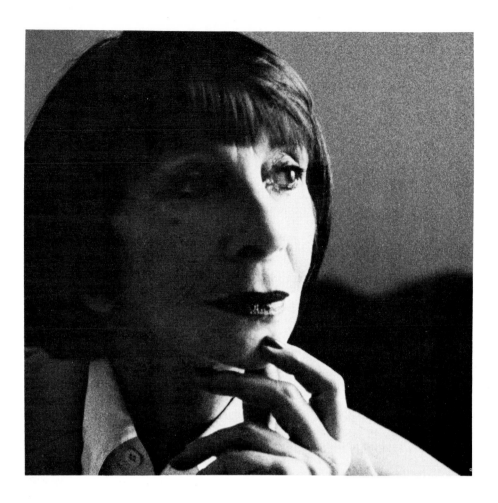

Introduction

There is no need for any young girl to have a shapeless body, for any mother to lose her figure after childbirth, or any mature woman to have an old and decrepit body.

If you want to always keep a young, youthful figure, you can – but to achieve this you must make exercise a way of life, and practise every day, every week, every month of the year.

It is true that everything worthwhile in life is worth working hard for, and surely it is worth a little hard work to achieve a super shapely body that walks well, a body on which clothes fall more beautifully, a body full of vitality that makes men aware, and makes you feel so happy to be alive.

Lotte Berk

Profile of Lotte Berk

When you first meet Lotte Berk, you notice her black hair, shining with a rich, deep gloss, and her dark eyes bright with mischief. When she demonstrates her exercises with swift, nimble agility you envy her shapely legs and slim, youthful figure of 34-24-35½. Petite and attractive, her whole personality is alive with a magnetism that cannot fail to attract you.

Lotte is truly a physical, sensual woman, who has attracted men throughout her life – seven times married, twice on paper, with a hundred lovers in between. Looking back, Lotte feels it was her earlier insecurity and constant need for the stimulation of new love, sex and new happenings, that drew her from one love affair to the next. Each new love, taking her into the different worlds of painters, musicians and dancers – each phase bringing a new circle of friends that reads like a 'Who's Who' of the artistic world.

When Lotte chatters gaily about her life, flitting quickly from one escapade to the next, you cannot fail to relish the taste of the drama, excitement and passions that make her life so rich.

She recalls her early career in modern ballet, when at eighteen she danced for the cream of conductors and producers, Bruno Walter, Fritz Busch and Carl Ebert, at the famous Salzburg Festival in Austria. Then as an emigrant, persecuted by the Nazis for being a Jew, she left behind a decadent era in Germany, and came to England – outrageous and blasé. 'In those early days in England, life was hard. Our escape from Germany had left us penniless. We found one room near Edgware Road, my husband Ernest and I slept on the floor, our baby daughter slept in the suitcase, and Mimi, my maid, in the bed. No work, no money, and I couldn't speak English!'

A bleak situation, enough to make most people give up hope. But Lotte – a survivor – fought back, loving the excitement and drama of building a completely new life. After a year of tremendous struggle, Lotte was discovered by Madame Rambert. She graced the stage at Covent Garden and was acclaimed as a great dancer in modern ballet.

'But as any dancer knows, operas and musicals don't run forever. When the show is finished it's back to auditions and the search for new work. I loved dancing and needed the money, so I took anything I was offered from low-brow to high-brow. From night-clubs, which I hated, to musicals and operas, which I loved. I adored dancing at the Glyndebourne and Edinburgh Festivals, and was most happy when I gave my own recitals.'

'Life then, in the 1930s was so full. I was never bored. I went to lots of parties, art balls at the Suffolk Gallery, and practically lived in the Café Royal, which was then *the* place for young artistes. In those days anyone who looked foreign, a bit different, was either laughed at or loved. Me? I was loved. Although I was not beautiful I seemed to attract men, and feeling so insecure I usually reacted to their flattery and attention.'

Eventually Lotte's need for love overtook her need for dancing, when at last an all-consuming love, so precious and wonderful, drew her away from the stage. But this, her greatest love, became her greatest tragedy. The end was so sad that Lotte will never talk about it. Anything else she will happily disclose, but this chapter of her life must remain untold.

For five months Lotte shut herself away. In solitude she read the five volumes of *Psychological Commentaries* by Maurice Nicoll and from his works found a feeling of contentment and security that changed her life.

From that tragedy Lotte's spirit fought back once more. She revived her life by moving in a new direction – with twenty years experience in modern ballet she dedicated her life to teaching women the art of obtaining a beautiful figure through exercise.

Then fate struck once more. An accident locked her lumbar spine and X-rays showed she would be crippled for life. Lotte refused to accept it – she exercised, and exercised, and exercised her back until just fourteen days later she proudly walked into her doctor's surgery. Her indomitable strength and spirit had triumphed again!

Life then 'took-off' once more. With the addition of orthopaedic movements, Lotte restyled her exercises and devised her unique method which is so famous today. In all walks of life Lotte is now acclaimed as the greatest woman in the field of physical fitness. To her pupils she is something very special – 'She applies her great knowledge of the body with a lot of human understanding' and they call her 'little boss'.

Her flat reflects her zany personality. The bathroom is covered with hand-painted murals. Tigers hover above the mirror waiting to pounce. Tropical birds fly over the ceiling, and luscious tempting fruit fight for your attention, alongside exotic plants. This painted paradise spills out into the bedroom and winds its way over the wall, leaving enough room for a mass of paintings by famous artists.

The original shopaholic – she buys expensive clothes to relieve a spate of boredom and nips around London in a racy custom-built black mini, complete with brown corduroy interior to match her eyes, and gold insignia 'LB' on the door.

Still sexy and sensual–'given a chance, sex and mischief never die' says Lotte as the beautiful men still lurk in the wings. 'It's strange, but all my life I feared that one day I would be alone. But now, with a deeper understanding of life, I have inner peace and am quite happy to live alone in my flat. In fact I find the freedom fantastic!'

'Although I feel that fundamentally we don't change, the works of Maurice Nicoll have taught me inner awareness. I now know that to give true happiness you must first look after your own happiness. If you can understand this, without thinking I'm conceited, then you know that it is very hard work to find true happiness alone.'

Emotionally Lotte has changed, but physically she's still the same. She once danced in Peter Pan as Tiger Lily, but now (born in 1913) she still bubbles and lives the part of the modern Peter Pan, with the petite shapely body – and energies – of a young woman. Lotte is truly unique. At sixty-five she looks forty-five. Sexually she is twenty-five. Deep within she feels eighteen – and holds the secret of youth.

Lotte Berk in Action

My first week with Lotte Berk will always be a vivid memory.

After a two-hour journey from the coast, I approached her studio in London with nervousness. I had heard so much about Lotte's method of exercise, and being extremely unfit I wondered if I could survive. But the promise of a slimmer figure, renewed vigour and vitality, together with a feeling of being 'so alive' rang in my ears. So what if it was hard work? The fulfilment of Lotte's promise must surely make it all worthwhile.

I arrived halfway through a lesson and was told to hang on the wall bar. 'We always start by "hanging" to loosen and stretch the spine' said Lotte, and trotted off to continue teaching a pupil her exercise. So I climbed the bars and 'hung'. My arms felt as though they would leave my shoulders, but determined not to look soft I hung on desperately. After several minutes, shrieks of laughter. 'Oh my God' said Lotte, 'you're only meant to hang for a few seconds!' But Lotte and her teachers soon made up for this by close attention throughout the lesson. (At times I wished they would forget about me again!)

The next session starts, the music plays and everyone does a lively programme of warm-up exercises. Stand tall, legs apart, arms above the head, swing up and down, up and down, swing through the legs, up and back, now arch the spine, bend forward and hold, touch the floor – keep legs straight! Up once more . . . The blood begins to pump through my veins as we stretch the waist, loosen the shoulders, firm the bosom, and loosen the neck.

As we warm-up (I feel as though I'm over-heating!) Lotte chats gaily with an effervescence that is contagious. Lotte loves astrology. 'When were you born?' she asks. 'December 14th' I reply. 'Ah! Sagittarius!' she exclaims. I wonder what thoughts lay behind that 'Ah!' Does she know the Sagittarian woman? – slightly clumsy, large appetite, likes good food and wine!

Linda Goodman describes the Sagittarian woman as 'the girl who strides down the street like a thoroughbred horse. You think she's the most graceful woman you've ever watched – until she stumbles on a crack in the sidewalk, awkwardly grabs the awning over the fruit stand to catch her balance and upsets two crates of oranges.'

Does Lotte know this? I wonder if she thinks I'm a hopeless case? No time to ponder. Warm-ups finish and the class moves to the barre. Like a ballet rehearsal we stand in a line along the wall.

'Bounces first' says Lotte, and she's in position before I've even moved. 'Squat on your feet, heels clicked together, knees open wide. Come up an inch. Hold. Up an inch more. Hold. Down an inch. Hold. What time of day were you born?' asks Lotte – she always asks questions in the middle of an exercise! Is it sadistic pleasure or a test of strength? 'Push the pelvis forward and stand up.' I stagger to an upright position and groan. Down again, this time legs together and small fast bounces. Lotte counts to thirty. I collapse after eight.

Only a few minutes gone and I'm already feeling muscles that I didn't know I had. 'Just wait until tomorrow' says a pupil with feeling. 'Then you'll know you've got them!'

The exercises continue at a fast pace – the class splits, 'Hanging bottoms or stomach?' asks Lotte. I need help for both, but choose stomachs. We lie on our backs. 'Relax the part God gave you for pleasure' says Lotte. One pupil relaxes her head and shoulders. 'God did not give you that for pleasure! Relax your pelvis.'

Now we are shown how to 'roll-in' the spine. Lotte demonstrates – it looks so easy. I sit up, hold onto my thighs and try to roll my spine into the floor. 'Slowly, one vertebra at a time, now tilt the pelvis.' My pelvic area seems rigid, my back straightens and 'I'm out'. Lotte tries an easier variation. I know what she wants me to do but my pelvis has a mind of its own. I try again. I'm still 'out'. I feel hopeless and exhausted, the sweat breaks out, but Lotte's patience is endless.

I join in on 'hanging bottoms'. Lois, Lotte's assistant takes over. 'Face the barre, right leg back, bend left knee, tilt the pelvis forward. Lift the right leg.

Hold. Bend stretch the right leg. Bend stretch. Bend stretch higher. (I've reached my limit, but still they ask.) Higher. Stretch the toes. Higher. Bend the right knee a little, lean over the leg. (I can't – my body wants to go the other way!) Now pull up. Hold it up. Up an inch. Roll the hip forward more. Pull the leg up higher. Relax!'

At least I'm not alone in the groans that follow.

On to the next exercise. I struggle to keep up. My brain hears the instructions but my body doesn't respond, and I'm doing weird movements completely out of time with everyone else.

Lotte laughs at my face, screwed up with concentration and suffering. 'Like a squashed lemon' she jokes. Her humour flows through the class. Like the artist she is, she outshines us all. The studio is her little theatre, and we pupils are her audience.

The class ends – the forty-five minutes are up (it seemed like a lifetime to me) and my legs feel like jelly. I leave the basement studio and my heart sinks as I face the stairs. The street seems a million miles up. Like a true Sagittarian I clumsily haul myself up by the railings and hobble home with a funny unbalanced feeling as if I've just stepped off a roller-coaster.

The next day is agony. My whole body seems to ache, it hurts to laugh, my legs are sore, going upstairs is hell and coming down again is worse!

I think of cookery writer Pru Leith, who told me that she had ridden horses for years and assumed she was fit. 'But twenty minutes of Lotte Berk turned my legs to jelly!' Suddenly I didn't feel so alone.

Two days later I'm back for another 'session'. Lotte shows me some more exercises to strengthen the stomach. We lie on our backs, knees bent, 'roll-in' the spine, reach up and relax. Five times more and Lotte asks where it hurts. 'Across my neck' I say – I seem to hurt in all the wrong places! 'Don't worry' says Lotte, 'that stiffness will go when your stomach gets stronger.' She helps me to relax my neck, and it's on to the next exercise. The class proceeds at the same lively pace, and I feel weaker than when I first started. Lotte assures me 'that's quite normal. For the first month you will feel exhausted (how true!) then you will master the movements and grow stronger. By the end of the third month you will be hooked and find that you can't live without exercise'.

By the end of twelve lessons, I feel I've improved a fraction and can now see why Lotte says it takes a year to get a lazy body into peak condition. Slowly I get a hint of feeling more alive. I walk away from the studio, no longer hobbling, but with a spring in my step. I feel refreshed instead of exhausted. A tingle of vitality seeps through my body and the Lotte promise of renewed vigour and health rings in my ears. I'm hooked!

Food and Slimming

How your body feels is important. It is governed by the way you feed it – remember that you are what you eat. So eat well and be healthy.

Vegetarianism is a sensible and healthy way of life, because the harrowing truth is that, today, few animals escape the barrage of chemicals (synthetic hormones, antibiotics, and insecticides) used in modern farming. After spending life on this chemical feast they are given tranquillisers prior to slaughter, then offered for your meal table.

It is impossible for animals to throw off all these chemicals, so the residue of accumulated toxins is passed on to you. While toxins do not produce sudden death, they do slowly poison the body – can anyone deny that these chemicals are likely to lead to illness and slow deterioration of the body?

Of course many people enjoy their roast beef with gravy – so if you feel you cannot give up meat try to reduce it to once or twice a week. You will also feel a benefit if you change from white and bleached food to wholemeal bread, unpolished brown rice and natural foods which are much tastier and so much better for you.

There are many good books on the market full of information on meatless protein and vegetarian food, so anyone wanting to change to a healthier way of eating can find plenty of ideas on meals and whole-food cooking.

If you want to lose weight quickly, for a holiday or special evening out, never be tempted to try a starvation diet. You will make yourself ill, and will probably eat twice as much afterwards, regaining any weight you have lost.

For a healthy person, a vegetable and fruit diet for three days will do no harm. Make up a variety of raw salads using any vegetables in season – cauliflower, grated carrots, spring onions, radishes, cucumbers, spinach, grated raw brussels, sliced mushrooms etc., then eat this freely at mealtimes with any fresh fruit (except bananas).

This will give you an initial weight loss of several pounds and is marvellous for cleansing the system. If you've been eating meat and commercial food products, you may experience headaches on the first day of this diet. This is a sign that your body is ridding itself of accumulated toxins, and whilst the headaches may not be pleasant, you will feel much better afterwards.

After three days on raw vegetables and fruit, continue with a well-balanced calorie controlled diet, keeping to within 1000–1200 calories a day.

To lose weight you must exclude all forms of sugar and flour, including ice-cream, sweets, cakes, biscuits, and pastries. Mayonnaise should be excluded, and French dressing limited to within your calorie allowance.

If you include nuts and cheese in your reducing diet, remember that nuts are 170 calories per ounce and cheddar cheese is 120 calories per ounce, so weigh these carefully and only allow yourself 1oz. of nuts or 1½ozs. of cheese at mealtimes. A jacket potato is only twenty-two calories per ounce, so a medium 5oz. potato could be included for only 110 calories – but be careful of the butter you add (two teaspoons of butter would be 100 calories). Calories do mount up quickly, so get a calorie booklet and carefully work out your daily allowance.

When you have reached your target weight, find out the calorie level at which you can maintain that weight, and keep to within your limit. A young girl can usually maintain weight on 1500 calories a day, but a woman over fifty must not exceed 1200 calories a day.

Although Lotte burns up a lot of energy – spending every morning in her studio – she still keeps within 1200 calories a day to maintain her teenage figure. She starts each day with a glass of warm water to cleanse the stomach. Breakfast is usually wholemeal toast, perhaps an egg, then coffee sweetened with honey. At lunch it's often just fruit – sometimes a banana with chopped nuts. Mid-afternoon, coffee with honey, and in the evening a light protein meal with salad or vegetables.

Most evenings Lotte indulges in her passion for fruit and often picks her way through a pound of grapes. She truly believes in eating healthy natural food with lots of fruit and vegetables. When she entertains you to lunch, she presents you with just a bowl of fruit – two apples and a banana – 'that's 180 calories, marvellous for the figure!'

Whether you are dieting or maintaining weight, Lotte says enjoy yourself.

'Don't make life hell. If you have a weight problem, then of course you must be careful what you eat. But allow yourself a treat now and again – treats make life fun! And if you want the odd alcoholic drink, why not! Even on a strict diet you could allow yourself a glass of dry wine (eighty calories). And if you "sin" and have a great cream bun at lunch, enjoy it – but balance it out by substituting dinner for some low-calorie fruit.'

Slimming, like exercise, is hard work. It needs determination, but those who learn to say 'no thank-you' find that all the effort is well rewarded. For losing weight means more than just being able to wear a belt or tucking in your blouse, it can give you that intangible, but so exciting *something* which is so valuable – CONFIDENCE.

N.B.   Before starting any diet, or any form of strenuous exercise, it is important to consult your doctor.

Why Exercise is so Important

The comparison of a human body to a motor car is overworked, but nevertheless it is still very valid. Think of a motor car that is left standing or used just once a week; gradually the parts seize up, the engine dries out, and its performance deteriorates. Then remember that all cars have a running-in period to allow the bearings to settle smoothly into their sockets and not jar out of alignment.

The human body is an even more intricate piece of machinery than any car, so the comparison emphasises the importance of regular exercise every day to keep the body in peak condition – a jog or game of squash once a week is not enough! And never start strenuous exercise if you have been madly inactive for a long time, start slowly, loosen up your muscles and gradually build up to harder exercises.

Dr Guy Beauchamp, leading manipulative surgeon in Harley Street, London has a good motto 'If you do not use it, you lose it'. He says 'This is true of fortune, friendship, love and health, and especially true in my field of physical medicine, which deals with the locomotion and joint movement. Unless joints are moved, unless fixation is caused to disappear, difficult mechanical problems arise. When accidents occur, particularly those which are common throughout the world – the whiplash injury to the neck, a strain through the mid or lower back – they often present symptoms which can be relieved by physical means. The treatment by exercise to obtain full mobility should be done every day, each week, each month, each year, and all one's life.'

As you get older your muscles tend to get shorter. With inactivity this contraction causes stiffness, aches and pains. But all this can be avoided by exercises which keep the muscles strong, supple and stretched. Regular practice of even simple exercises is an absolute necessity. They help to prevent the onset of many minor complaints – tension, headaches, fatigue and insomnia. Rheumatism, lumbar pains and backache can also be eased with movements that loosen the joints, and depression and psychosomatic complaints can be relieved through exercises that stimulate the adrenalin glands – a regular shot of adrenalin is a wonderful cure for lethargy and boredom!

In pregnancy, a little light exercise is also beneficial, although many of the exercises in this book are too tough for a pregnant woman. If you are really fit you could do the leg and thigh exercises, but Lotte says 'Why not enjoy your pregnancy (be careful not to overeat!) and then start exercising quickly after the birth to regain your figure. Six weeks after childbirth is the ideal time to start.'

In conjunction with dieting, exercise is most important. How many women have successfully lost their fat and still been dissatisfied with a body soft like butter? And for those who don't need to diet, how many times have we heard the words of despair – 'My hips are only thirty-six inches but my thighs stick out at the top . . .' 'I am bottom heavy and no matter how I try, cannot slim down my hips. If I go on a diet, I only lose it from my bust . . .'

The answer to this kind of problem is exercise, and with the exercises in this book you can improve your figure – cure bulging thighs, sagging stomachs, drooping bottoms and shapeless waistlines. Based on modern ballet, yoga and orthopaedics, these exercises will stimulate the heart, glands and hormones, get the adrenalin flowing and help the body to sweat naturally to excrete accumulated toxins. So you also gain from the health-giving benefits of stimulating exercise.

One pupil who has found the rewards from Lotte's method of exercise is Janine Ingram, designer for Harold Ingram knitwear, who happily tells of the change it has made in her life. 'Lotte's method of exercise has helped me change from an awkward hefty woman into a supple slim girl. The feeling of being fit and slim is marvellous, but more than that, I've regained my *joie de vivre* after a cancer operation, by being fitter than I ever was before.'

The list of people who value the importance of exercise and flock to Lotte's studios is endless: Barbara Ferris, Lee Remick, Carol Linley, Yolande Donlan, Joan Collins, Beverley Sassoon, Barbra Streisand and Britt Ekland. Secretaries and housewives flock there too, and at Lotte's studio age is no limit. Pupils of fifty and over prove that exercise is not just a kid's game – it's for a lifetime.

So if you are fifty plus and feeling stiff, please don't think it is too late to start exercising. It is never too late. Everyone can benefit from the exercises in this book.

How to Use This Book

First of all, make up your mind that you will do some exercises *every* day, because a regular daily session is most important if you want to have a super figure. It really is no good to do an hour's exercise the first day, relax for a week, then another spurt of exercises, and so on . . . This way you will achieve nothing. Even ten minutes exercise once a day is better than an hour once a week, although ideally a regular twenty-minute session would be best.

Some people prefer to do their exercises in the morning, but if you are rushing to go to work, you could do your exercises in the evening – but never immediately after a heavy meal. Choose the best time for you and make up your mind that exercise is going to become a part of your daily life.

Start by carefully reading each exercise and study the photographs. Then, if possible, practise in front of a mirror, checking once again with the photographs, to ensure that you are doing the movements correctly.

At first your muscles and limbs will ache and feel stiff – this is quite normal when you start to use muscles that haven't been used for years – but none of these exercises should hurt your spine. So if you feel a pain in the lumbar or lower back region, stop immediately, because you are doing the exercise wrongly. Re-read the instructions, study the pictures, and start again.

If you are exercising with a friend, then you can watch each other, checking the movements with the photographs and correcting any faults, until you have mastered each exercise correctly.

At first, you should work out a simple daily programme, beginning with the warm-up exercises, followed by the first two exercises in each section. Then as you get stronger you can progress to other exercises, varying your programme to suit yourself.

You will see that the exercises in this book have been arranged in sections for legs and thighs, stomach, bottom etc., so if you have any particular figure problem you can concentrate on the relevant exercises. But please read the notes prior to the warm-up exercises, and remember that you must always start each daily session with your warm-up routine.

Just start slowly, practise and master each exercise before you move on to the next, and *never* attempt to do all the exercises in the first week. If you are unfit you will find many of the exercises impossible, you'll feel deflated and will be in danger of giving up before you have even begun.

Yes, some of the exercises are hard, but don't try to make them easier by cheating! If we say the body must be straight, then it *must* be straight. Bending the body may make the movement easier (and less painful!) but you will lose the benefit of that particular exercise. Just remember that these exercises have been specially devised to work on lazy muscles and correct figure faults, so be tough on yourself, aim for perfection and you will be rewarded with the results.

Be dedicated – and be patient. If your muscles are lazy and your body is flabby, it will take time to tone and firm those muscles and improve your shape, so please do not expect results overnight. Just think that every day you are one step nearer to your goal. At first your waist will become slimmer, your skirts and trousers will become a bit looser, then your stomach will flatten and firm. If your thighs are a problem area, then you may have to exercise regularly for several months before you see results – the secret is to persevere.

And never look upon your exercises as a chore, a drudge that must be suffered, just think of them as a daily programme that will give you zest and vitality. If you are exercising with friends, then relax, make it a fun session and have a good laugh — and enjoy the wolf-whistles that will follow!

Choose some gay lively music that makes you feel good, and do all the exercises in rhythm with the music – just let your body flow and move as if you were dancing. At the moment, Lotte likes Abba, Donna Summers and pop music that creates a feeling of fun and laughter.

Wear something that allows you to move freely, without restriction – bra and panties are fine, but tights and a leotard do make you feel sleeker when you look at yourself in the mirror – you can even exercise in the nude if you like looking at yourself.

So now turn the pages and you will be ready to embark on the pathway to a beautiful body. This book will show you how to achieve that sexy shape, but be dedicated, because in the end, it is up to you to do it.

Warming Up

Warm-up exercises are an important part of your daily exercise programme. They act as a boost to your whole system – increasing circulation, pumping blood to the tissues, warming the muscles and loosening up the body ready for more specific exercise.

When exercising at home, remember that you must *always* start each session with your warm-ups and never go straight into concentrated exercises. 'Warm' muscles are loose and flexible, but 'cold' muscles can easily tear, so even if you only want to firm and flatten your stomach, don't be tempted to do just the stomach exercises – always start with the 'warm-ups' first.

In Lotte's studio, every session starts with the warm-up exercises, numbers 1–6, which are done as a lively continuous programme, without any pause in between. So as soon as you have learnt these exercises do the same at home – start with warm-up exercise 1, repeat ten times, go straight into exercise 2, repeat five times, let your movements flow into exercise 3 . . . and so on.

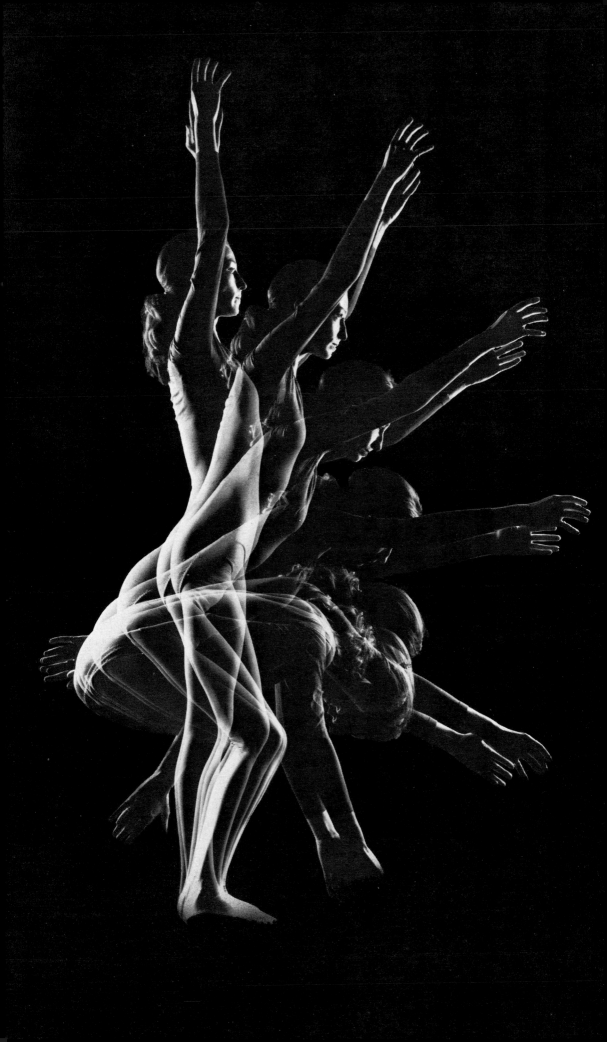

Exercise 1

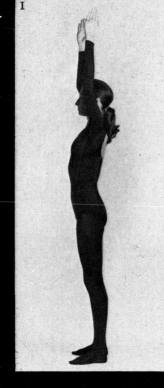

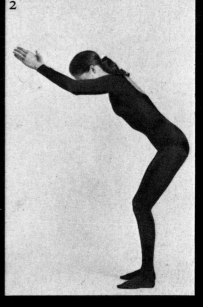

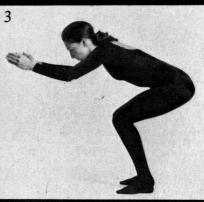

In Lotte's studio, at the start of each session, students 'hang' from the wall bars in order to stretch the spine. At home, you must also stretch the spine before exercising, just as a cat str-e-tches before leaping into action, so . . .

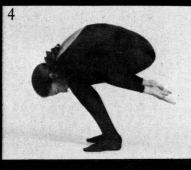

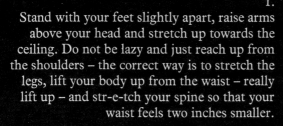

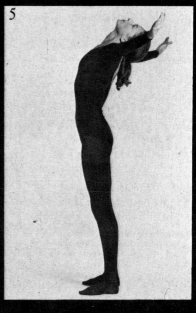

1.
Stand with your feet slightly apart, raise arms above your head and stretch up towards the ceiling. Do not be lazy and just reach up from the shoulders – the correct way is to stretch the legs, lift your body up from the waist – really lift up – and str-e-tch your spine so that your waist feels two inches smaller.

2–4.
Now bend your knees and swing your arms forwards, down towards the floor, and sweep them behind you.

5.
Keeping your feet flat on the floor swing your arms forwards, come up again, swinging your arms behind your head and bend the elbows.

Repeat from position 2, ten times, and just let your body flow into a continuous swing, up and down, up and down.

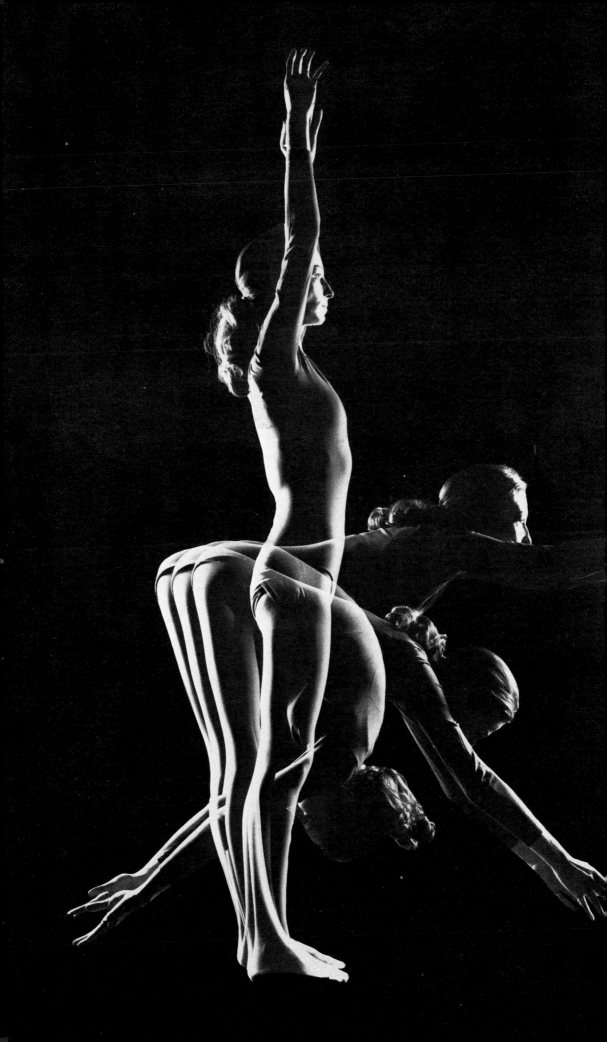

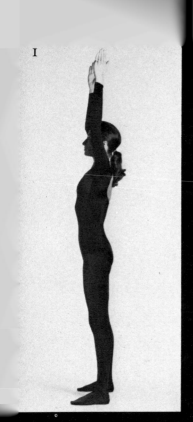

1

2

3

4

I.

tall with your feet wide apart
d stretch up as in Exercise I.

2.

Keeping arms and body in a
t line, push your bottom out,
ur spine, bend forward from
the hips and bring your body
parallel to the floor. Hold this
n for a few seconds, and keep
egs absolutely straight. If you
doing this correctly it should
urt at the back of your thighs.

3.

the body and touch the floor

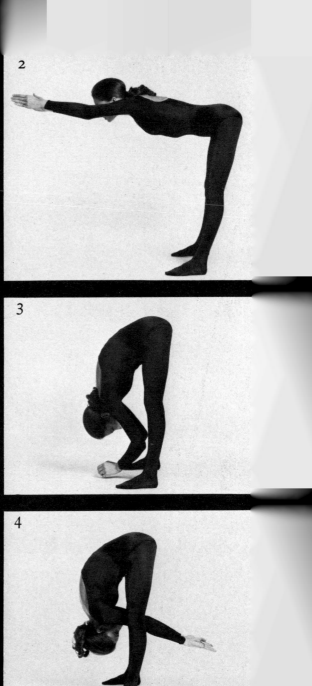

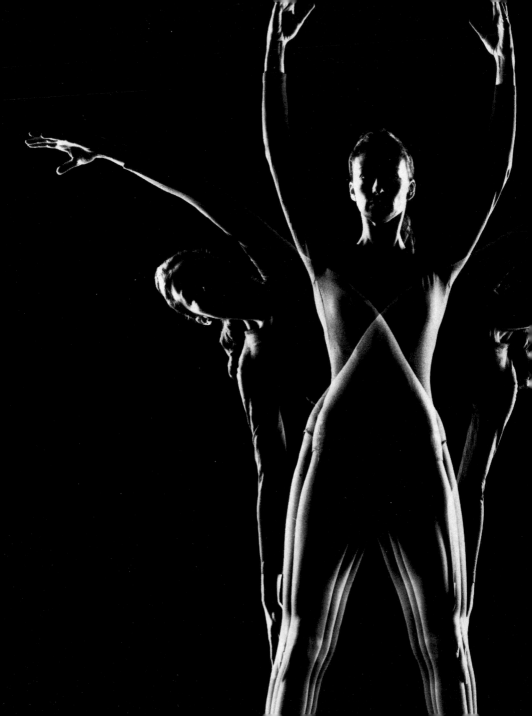

Exercise 3

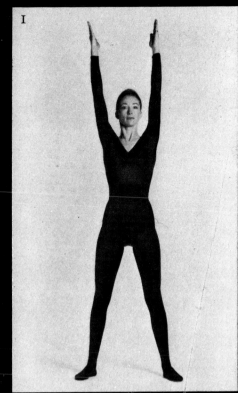

I.
Stand with your legs apart and stretch up tall.

2.
Keeping your legs straight, swing left arm over your head and slide your right arm down the right leg. Go over as far as possible, and *really* feel that pull in your waist.

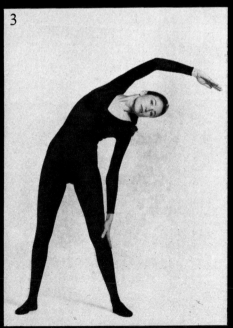

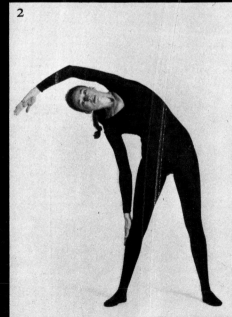

3.
Swing back to an upright position, and swing over the other side. Repeat positions 2 and 3 (ten times).

Do not cheat by leaning forwards. If possible, try and do this exercise sideways on to a mirror, and check that your legs, body and arms are all in line.

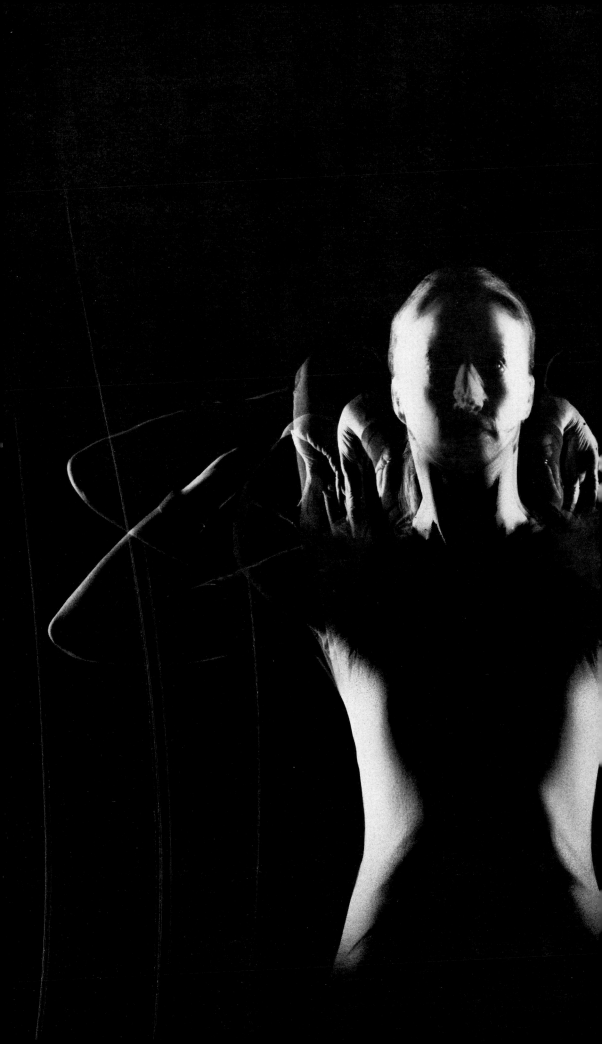

Exercise 4

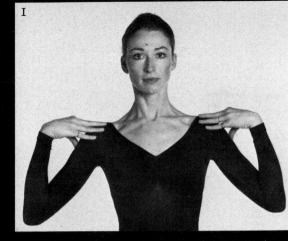

This exercise should be incorporated into your warm-up routine, but can also be done at any time to relieve rheumatic aches and stiffness in the shoulders.

1.
Stand tall, and place your hands on your shoulders.

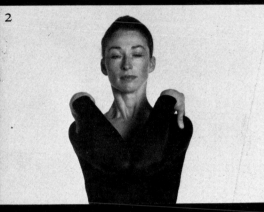

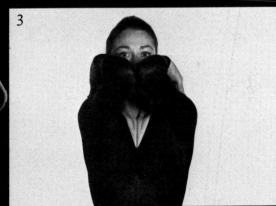

2–4.
Now make a circling movement with your elbows, by bringing the elbows down, forwards and together, then up, and circle them backwards.

Repeat eight times in a continuous movement, and make sure that you really push those elbows up high, and open them as wide as possible.

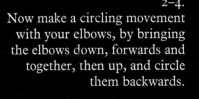

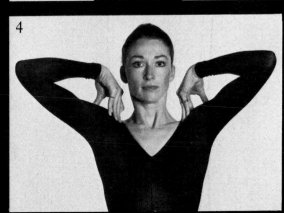

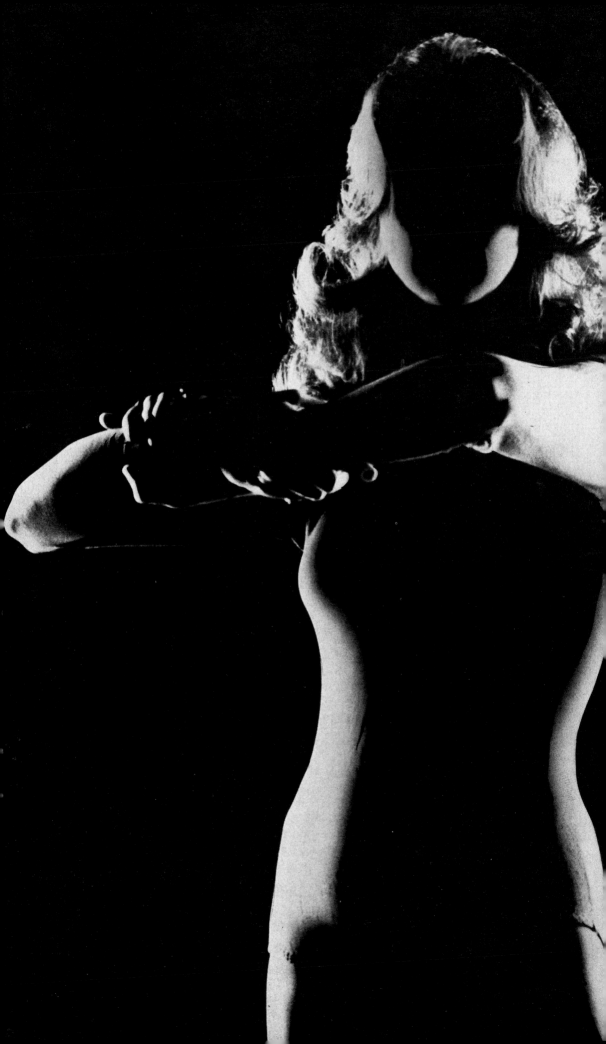

Exercise 5

Exercises cannot do very much to change the shape and size of your bust, as bosoms are determined by glands. But the muscles around the bosom can be tightened, and this will help to 'lift' a sagging bustline.

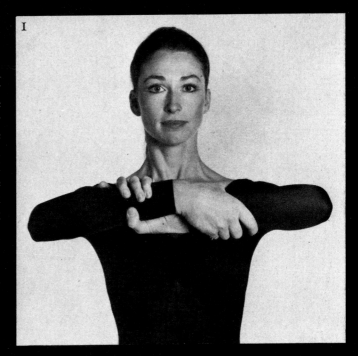

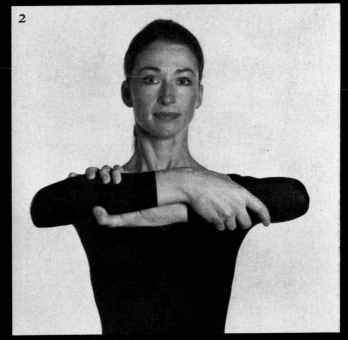

1.
Stand tall, cross your arms in front of breasts and grip your inner wrists.

2.
Without releasing this position, jerk your hands towards your elbows as if you were trying to push up your sleeves. Push and relax, push and relax. Repeat ten times.

Check this exercise in front of a mirror – if you are doing it correctly your breasts will jump up and down!

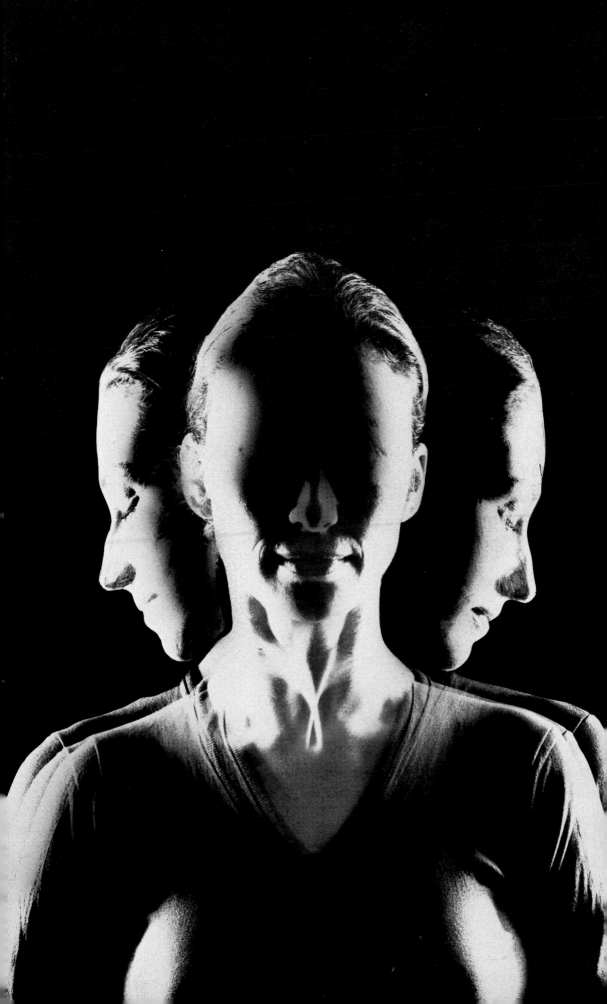

Exercise 6

These exercises are an important part of your daily warm-up routine, as they help to keep a youthful appearance – have you noticed how many older people turn their whole body to look while a young girl gracefully turns her neck!

You can also do these exercises at any time to release tension and stiffness in the neck.

1–3.
Stand tall, with head erect. Now bend your neck and push your left ear towards the left shoulder. You should really feel the pull in your neck! Bring your head up and bend your neck the opposite side. Repeat five times and remember to keep your head in line with your shoulders – do not let your head drop forwards.

4 & 5.
Twist your head and look to the left, then to the right. Try to push your chin towards each shoulder – but keep the shoulders still! Repeat five times.

6–10.
Twist your head and look over your left shoulder. Now relax the neck, roll your head forwards in a half-circle sweeping across your chest to look over your right shoulder. Reverse the swing from right to left and repeat five times.

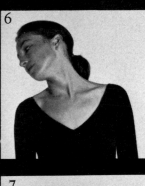

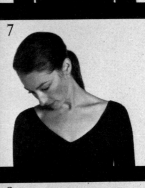

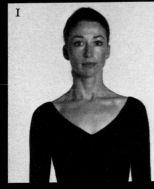

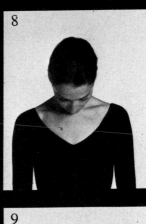

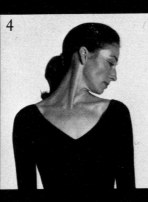

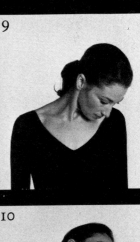

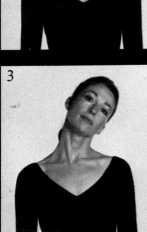

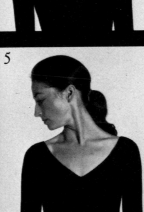

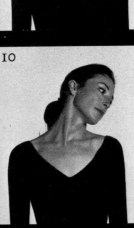

Legs and Thighs

Many women suffer with flabby thighs, and although exercises cannot actually take away fat, you can reshape your legs and make them thinner by firming and toning the muscles.

But first determine whether your muscles are just flabby or whether you are carrying excess fat by stretching your leg in front of you and 'pinching' the flesh on your thigh. An inch of spare flesh is normal, but if you can 'pinch' more than that, then you are overweight and must start dieting. If you just have flabby thighs, then you must start exercising.

Start today, and please don't give up when you see no improvement in a few weeks, because your thighs will take longest to shape. Go on with your exercises and be assured that the results *will* come.

The worst part of slimming your thighs is the initial agony that you will suffer when you start to exercise. You may even feel like resting for a few days until the ache subsides, but don't! Your aches will return again after the next session and you'll never progress. Even if your legs feel sore and stiff, you must keep up with your daily exercise programme; just start as usual with some gentle warm-up exercises, and you will find that as your circulation begins to flow, your muscles will loosen up and your aches will disappear.

If you are out of condition you may also get cramp in your feet, so just stamp your feet on the floor and again carry on with your exercising. Gradually as you improve, any tendency towards cramp will disappear.

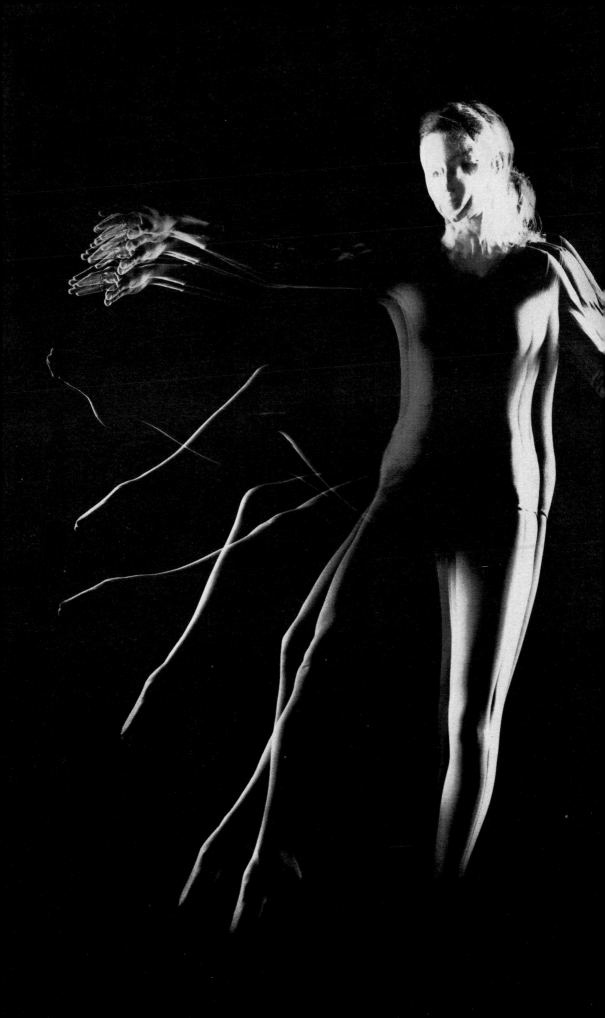

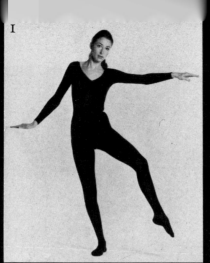

1

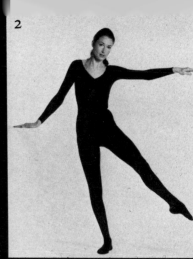

2

a
elf
d,
at
nt
ot
of
dy
eg.

1 & 2.
Bend your right knee and lift the leg a
few inches off the floor, then str-e-tch
the leg hard and point those toes!

3 & 4.
Bend the right knee again, lifting your
our leg as high as possible and stretch
the leg hard until it is really straight.

5.
Keeping the leg straight, pull your
foot towards you and lift your leg
higher. Keep leaning over that leg,
and use that lazy thigh muscle to lift
up-up-up-up . . . and you should be
in agony!

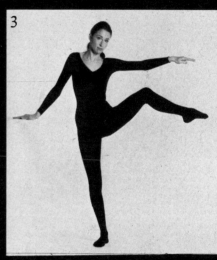

3

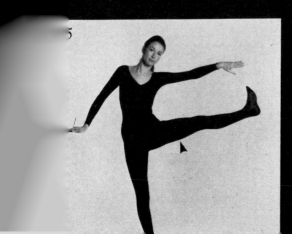

4

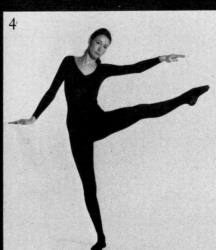

5

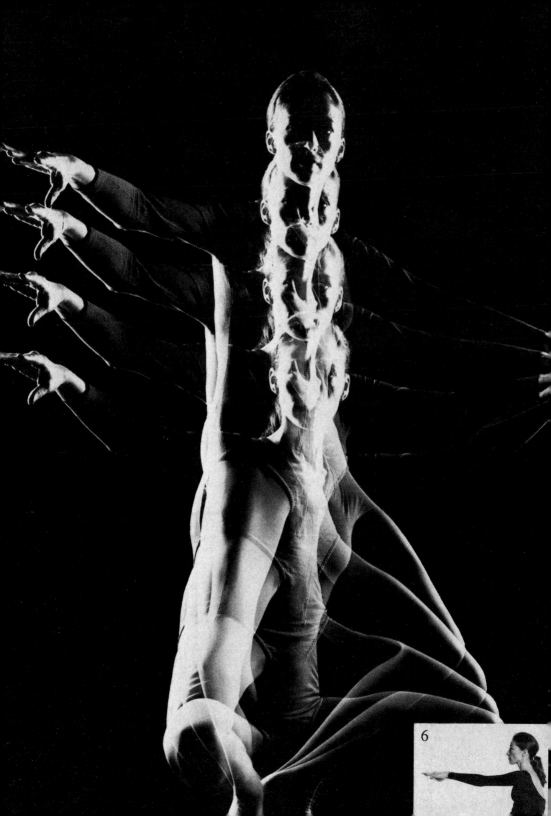

6

Exercise 8

There are three stages to this exercise, each working on a different part of your thigh muscles, giving you super all-round exercise to slim your legs into shape.

1.
Stand sideways to a chair, table or any firm object at waist level. Steady yourself with your left hand, hold your right arm at shoulder level and squat onto the balls of your feet. Your knees must be as wide apart as possible and your heels clicked firmly together.

2.
Now do small bounces up and down, keeping the back absolutely straight – do not lean forwards! Start with five bounces each day and gradually build up to forty. This movement works on the top and back of your thigh muscles.

3.
Keeping the same 'squat' position, with knees wide apart and heels clicked together, bring your body up so that your bottom is about a foot off the floor. Hold this position – keep your back straight – and push the knees open wider. Do little pushes open, open, open to the count of ten. Relax and repeat. This movement will get the inner and outer thigh muscles working.

4.
Now face the chair or table. Steady yourself with both hands, and with knees *together*, go down on tip-toes into your squat position.

5.
Keeping your back straight, lift the body a few inches off your heels.

6.
Now without moving the upper body, just push the pelvic bone forward. Hold to a count of three – you should feel the front thigh muscles working – and relax into your squat position. This is a tough movement, so try and start with five repetitions and build up to fifteen.

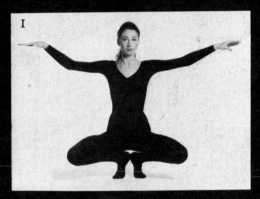

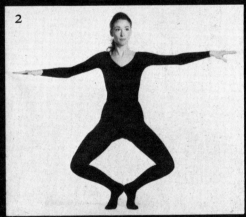

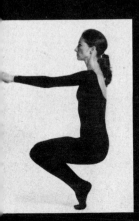

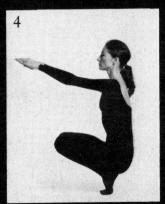

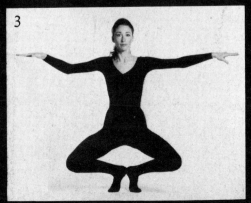

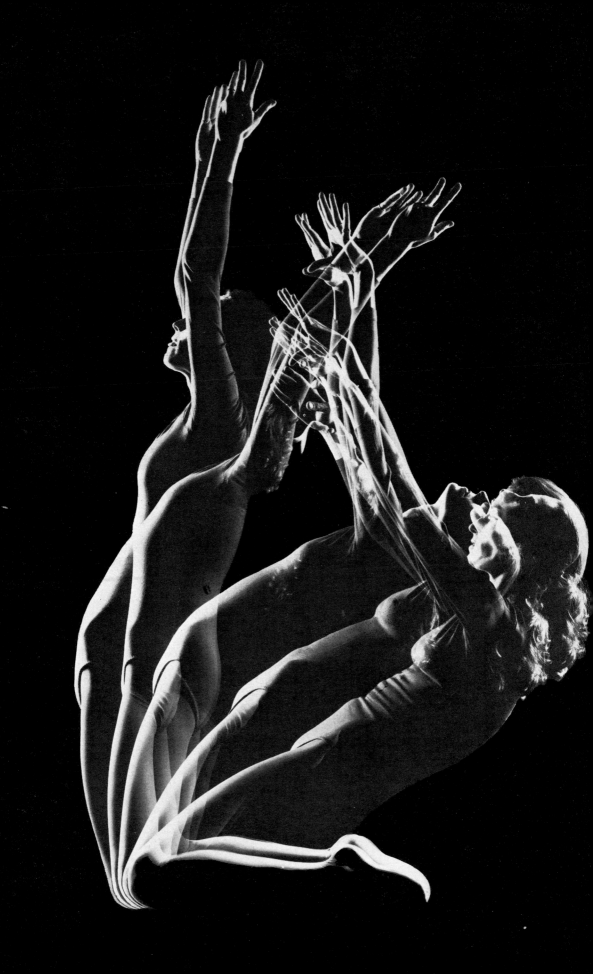

Exercise 9

I.
Kneel on a carpet with knees slightly apart, and lean backwards with your upper body slightly rounded forwards.

2–4.
Without moving your upper body, thrust the pelvic bone forwards from your hips, and push forwards until your thighs are upright to the floor. Follow through with your upper body, lift your arms, and bring your body upright.

Remember that you have got to get your pelvic bone and thighs completely forward, *before* you start to move your upper body.

Repeat three times and slowly increase to ten. As you get stronger you will be able to lean back lower on the starting position. The lower you go the more effective this will be on your thigh muscles.

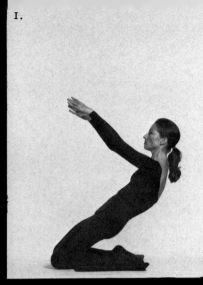

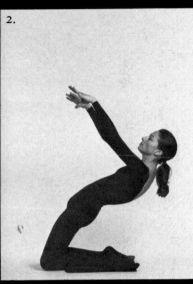

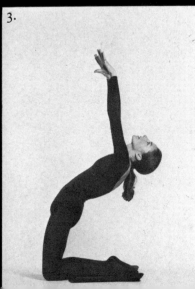

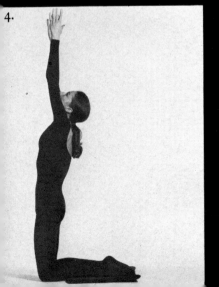

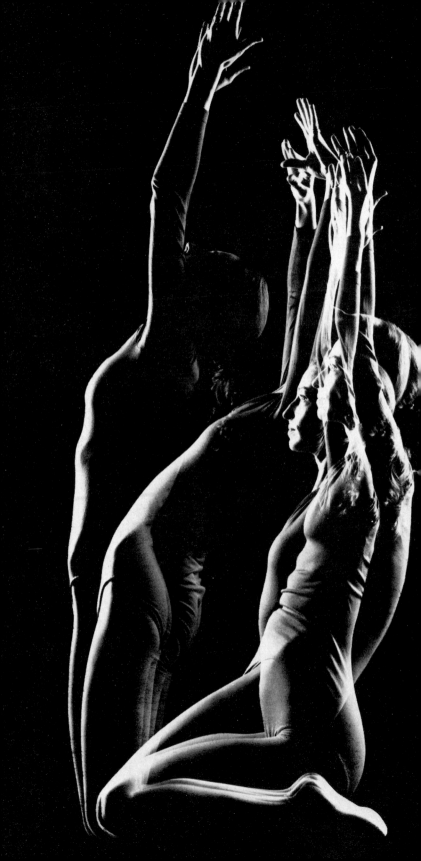

Exercise 10

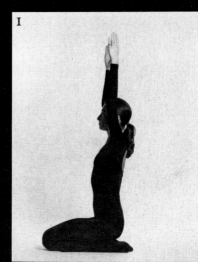

1.
Sit upright on your heels with knees together, raise arms above your head, and if possible check yourself in a mirror to make sure you are not leaning forwards.

2.
Keeping your arms and upper body still, 'click' the pelvic bone forward – this movement will lift the thighs and body – and hold this position for a count of three.

3 & 4.
Then using just the thigh muscles, slowly lift your whole body until you are in an upright position. Repeat three times.

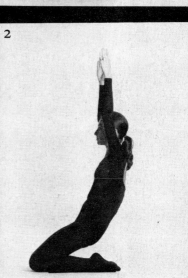

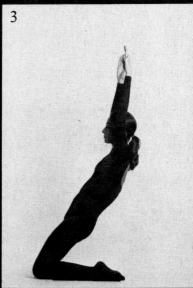

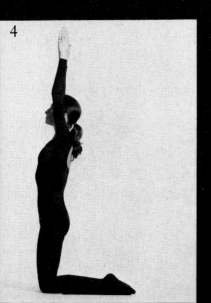

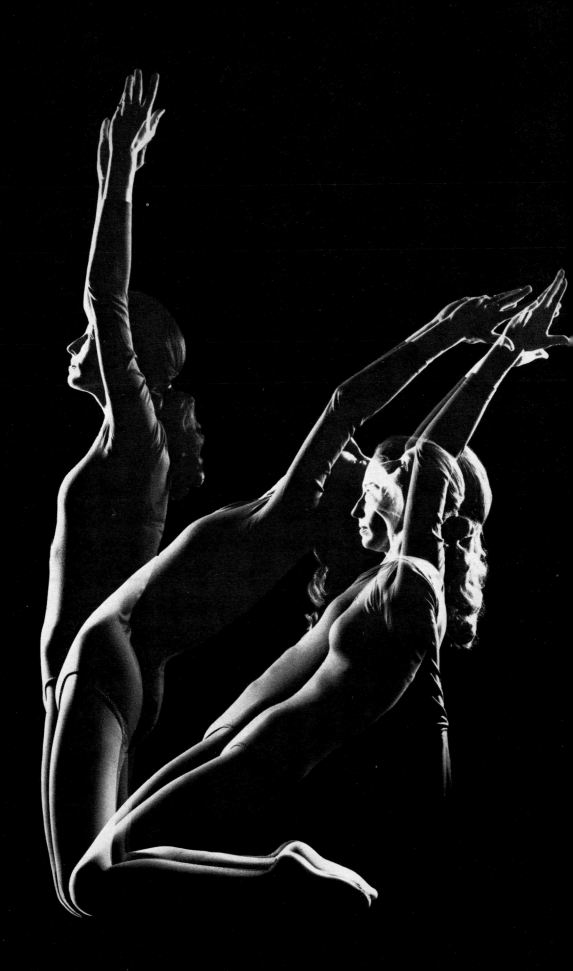

1.
Kneel on a carpet with knees about a foot apart and bring your feet slightly together. Lean back and place fingertips on the floor behind you, lean onto your fingers and raise your bottom so that your body is in a straight line.

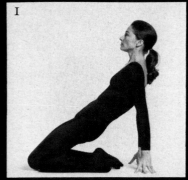

2 & 3.
Now raise your arms in the air – but do not let your body drop back! Your thigh muscles should support your body and keep it still.

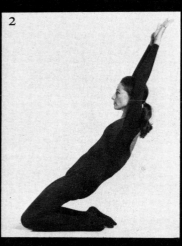

4 & 5.
Thrust your pelvic bone forward from the hips, push your thighs forward, follow through with your upper body and stretch up towards the ceiling. Relax and repeat.

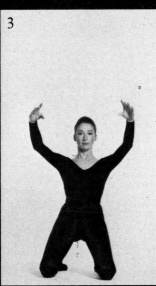
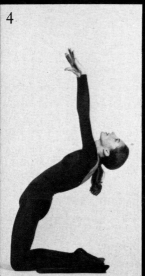
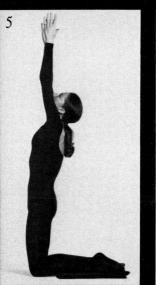

Exercise 12

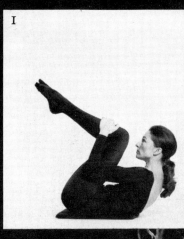

I

This exercise is for beginners with weak stomach muscles. If you are very weak you can start doing this exercise by 'walking' against a wall. Otherwise do this in the middle of a room without any support.

1.
Lie on a carpet on your back, curl your body round, bringing knees and head together.

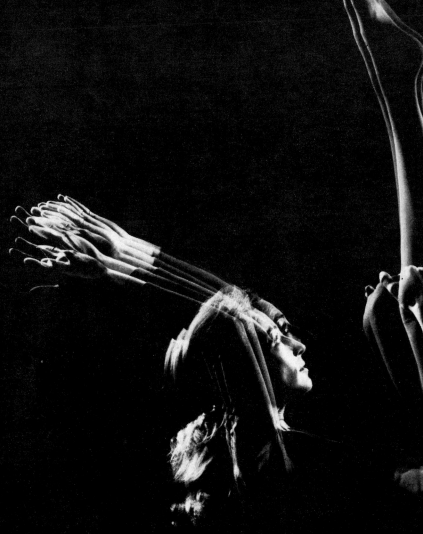

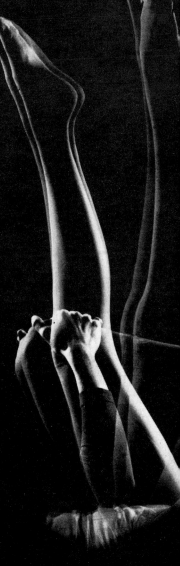

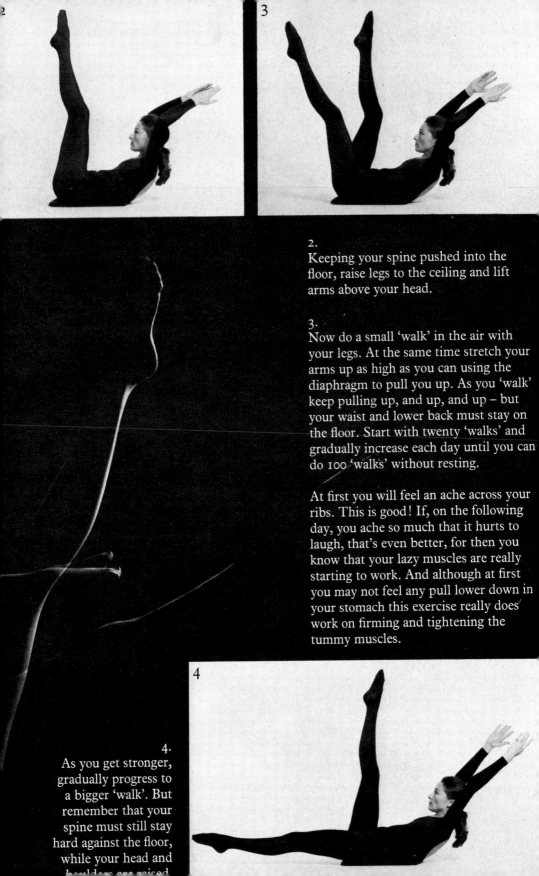

2

2.
Keeping your spine pushed into the floor, raise legs to the ceiling and lift arms above your head.

3.
Now do a small 'walk' in the air with your legs. At the same time stretch your arms up as high as you can using the diaphragm to pull you up. As you 'walk' keep pulling up, and up, and up – but your waist and lower back must stay on the floor. Start with twenty 'walks' and gradually increase each day until you can do 100 'walks' without resting.

At first you will feel an ache across your ribs. This is good! If, on the following day, you ache so much that it hurts to laugh, that's even better, for then you know that your lazy muscles are really starting to work. And although at first you may not feel any pull lower down in your stomach this exercise really does work on firming and tightening the tummy muscles.

4.
As you get stronger, gradually progress to a bigger 'walk'. But remember that your spine must still stay hard against the floor, while your head and

Stomach

The stomach muscles are never used in everyday life, which is the reason for too many shapeless waistlines. Even after a successful diet many women find they still have a soft flabby tummy, so these exercises will do what many diets cannot do – firm and flatten the stomach to give you a trim shapely body.

And for women who suffer from pre-menstrual cramps and pains, there's an added bonus. These exercises, when practised regularly, will release abdominal tensions and relieve monthly pains.

The first two exercises in this section – numbers 12 and 14 – are for beginners with very weak muscles. These exercises are also ideal for overweight people, and for mothers six weeks after childbirth, to start tightening the stomach muscles and regaining a trim figure.

Beginners should concentrate on these two exercises – but make sure you also understand the 'rolling-in' of the pelvis which is shown as exercise 13. Practise, practise and practise hard every day until your muscles are stronger and you have built up to the maximum number of repetitions. You will now be able to progress to the other exercises in this section and should already be seeing an improvement in your shape.

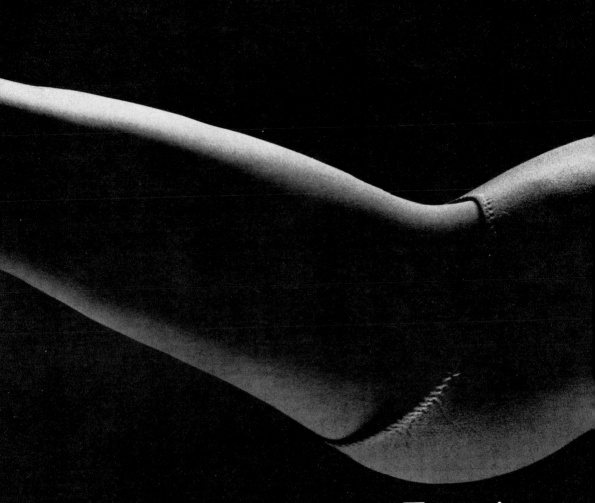

Exercise 13

Many of the following exercises are based on Lotte's unique method of 'rolling-in' the pelvis – she calls it her love-making position. It is important that you understand this movement, so practise several times before you move on to the following exercises.

1.
Lie on a carpet on your back, with knees bent. If you lie naturally, your spine will be arched and off the floor and you will be able to slide your hand under your spine. Try it and see.

2.
Now 'roll-in' the pelvis by pushing your spine flat against the carpet so that your bottom comes slightly off the floor. In this position you should not be able to slide your hand under the spine.

3.
To check that you are doing this movement correctly, look at your inner thigh muscles. Note their position when you are lying naturally and then see how they change when you 'roll-in' the pelvis. If done correctly, the inner thigh muscles will 'jump-out'.*

*See picture 3

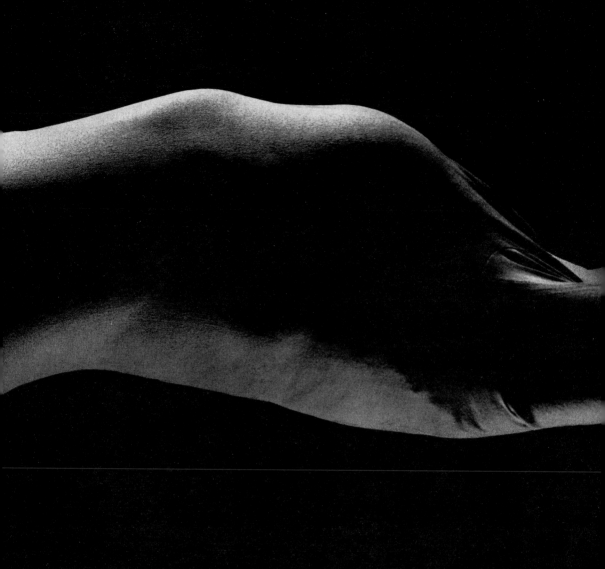

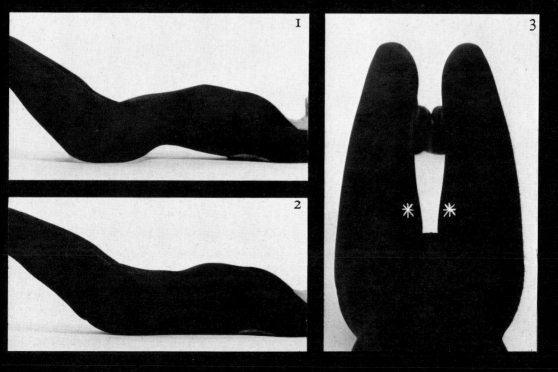

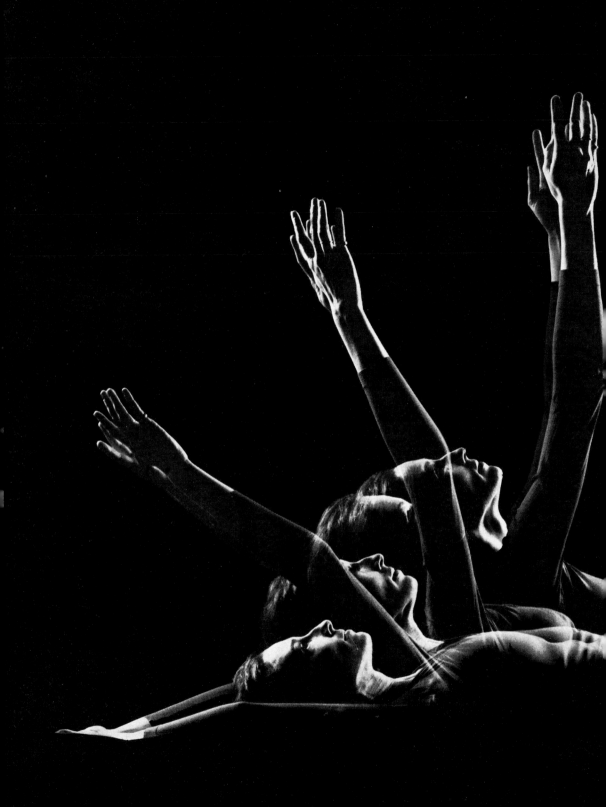

Exercise 14

This is another simple exercise for people with weak stomach muscles.

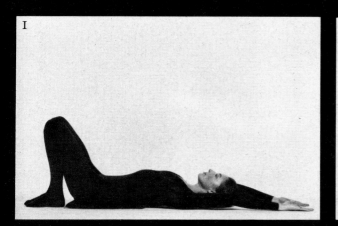

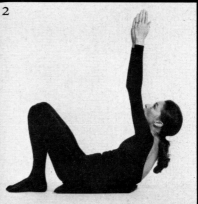

1.
Lie on a carpet on your back, bend knees, keeping feet flat on the floor and bring heels up close to your bottom. Stretch arms behind your head.

2.
Now 'roll-in' the pelvis, (concentrate on the movement and make sure you get it right) then lift arms, head and shoulders off the floor and stretch up hard. Stretch up and up – hold it – and relax.

Remember that your pelvis must remain 'rolled-in' and your waist must be hard on the floor when you lift and stretch up. Repeat the exercise fifteen times and build up to fifty.

Beginners with a weak stomach tend to strain from the neck when they stretch up, so if you feel any tension just shake your head loosely and try to relax the neck. But if you still get an ache across the shoulders, don't worry, this tension will go as your stomach muscles get stronger.

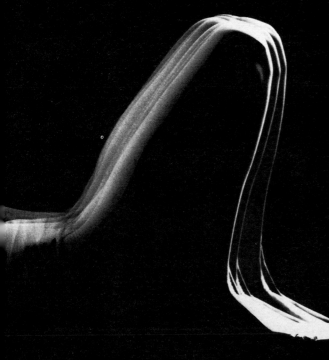

Exercise 15

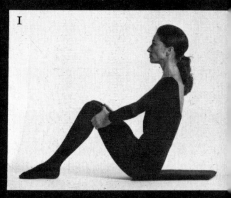

Beginners trying to perfect this exercise may find it easier by tucking their feet under the edge of a bed or settee, for extra support.

1.
Sit on the floor on a carpet, bend knees, hold on to your thighs and straighten your spine.

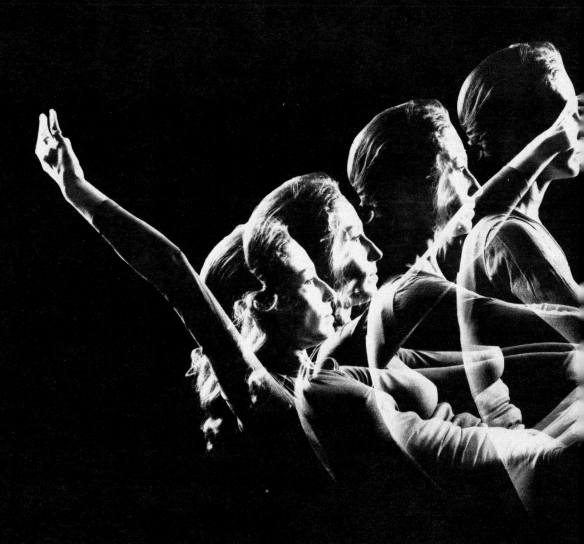

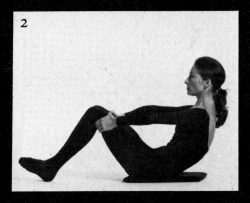

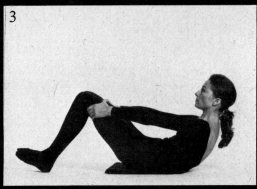

2.
Slowly push each vertebra into the floor, one by one. At this stage, *only* your pelvic area should be moving, so start by moving backwards from your hip joints. Beginners with a weak stomach may only get as far as this . . .

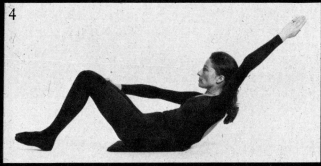

3.
And as you get stronger, you will be able to get your body lower, like this . . .

4.
Now lift one arm in the air – but your body must remain still – do not let it drop backwards. Gently curl the upper body over your waist in

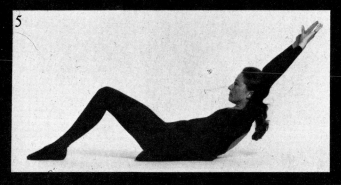

small bounces, by pulling gently with the hand holding your thigh. You should now feel a pull in your diaphragm.

If your pelvis lifts forward and your back straightens you have lost the movement. This often happens with beginners, but don't try and correct it, just go back to the beginning and slowly start again. Repeat six times.

5.
As you get stronger, you will be able to lift both arms off, (still with the pelvis rolled into the floor) then sit up and stretch up towards the ceiling.

Exercise 16

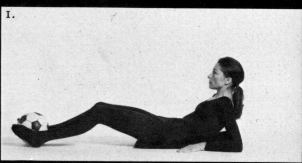

This is a fun exercise
that you can do at
home, or on the beach.

I.
Lie on your back on a carpet.
Support your upper body with your
elbows and hold a beach ball
between your feet.

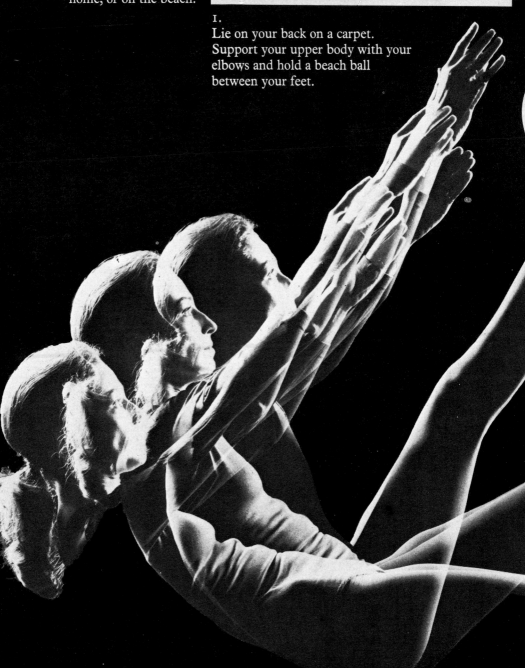

2.

Now 'roll-in' the pelvis, pushing waist hard against the floor, then lift arms above your head and at the same time lift the ball slightly off the floor.

Your waist *must* remain hard against the floor. If you find you arch your spine as you lift your arms up, then your stomach is not yet strong enough to do this exercise. Go back and concentrate on the previous stomach exercises and return to this when you are stronger.

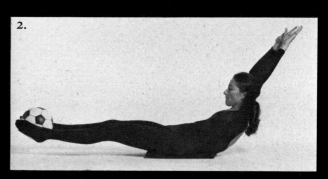

2.

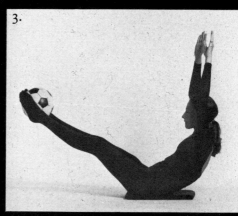

3.

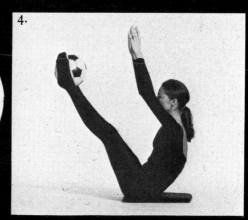

4.

3 & 4.
As you improve you will be able to lift the ball and your arms higher – and higher.

Exercise 17

This is an advanced exercise for pupils with strong
stomach muscles, so do not attempt this unless you can
do all the previous stomach exercises. Beginners
should not look upon this exercise as an impossibility
but accept this as a challenge, a goal to aim for.

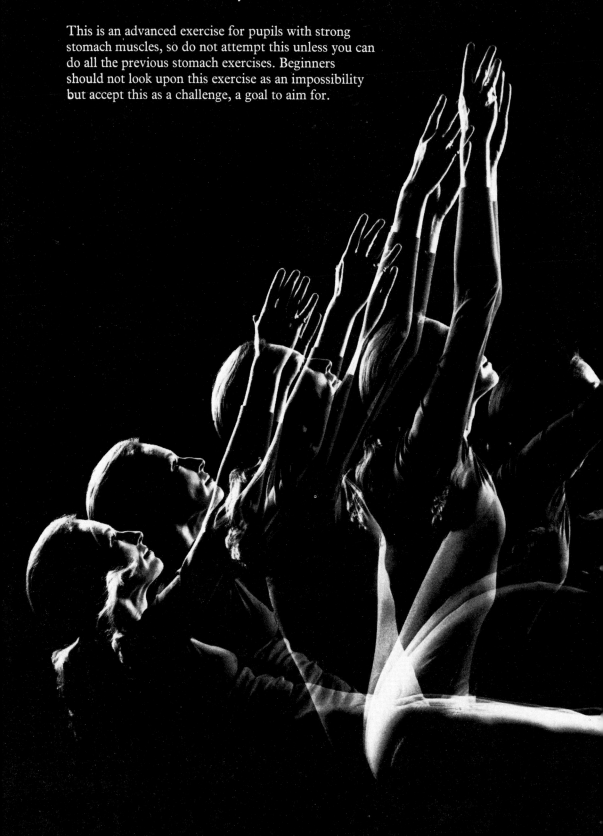

1.
Lie on a carpet on your back, legs together and arms stretched behind your head.

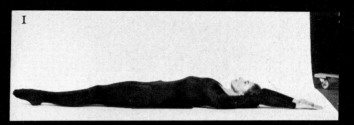

2.
Keeping your arms still, slowly lift your body off the ground, using just the stomach muscles to pull you up – don't cheat and whip your arms forward.

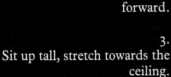
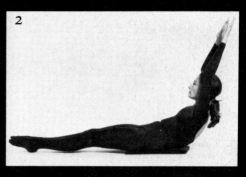

3.
Sit up tall, stretch towards the ceiling.

4.
Then bend forward from the hips, take hold of your feet and touch your knees with your head.

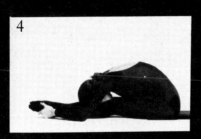

5.
As you get even stronger, you can do this exercise with your legs wide open.

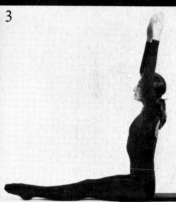

6.
As you bend forwards from the hips, you take hold of your toes, and touch the floor with your head.

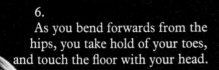
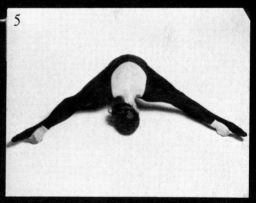

Wow! Now your stomach is truly strong and firm! Wasn't it worth all the hard work?

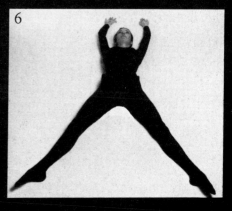

Exercise 18

This final stomach exercise is also tough, but when you are strong enough to accomplish this, you will have the reward of knowing that you have achieved perfection with your stomach muscles, and you will then be as fit, strong – and slim – as a dancer.

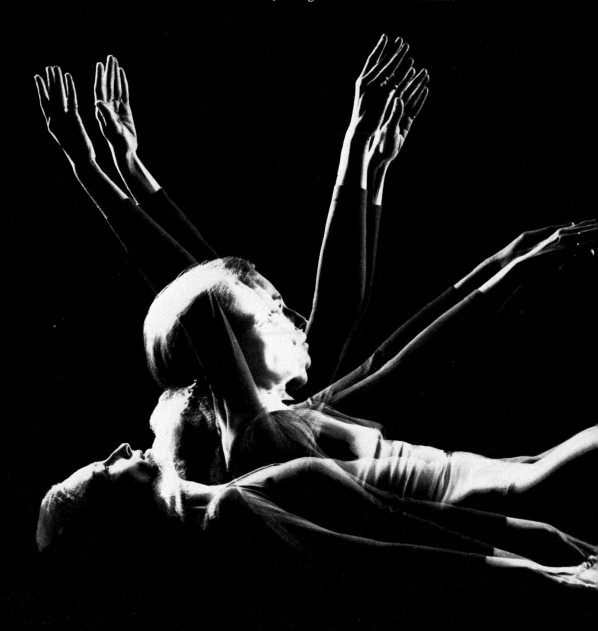

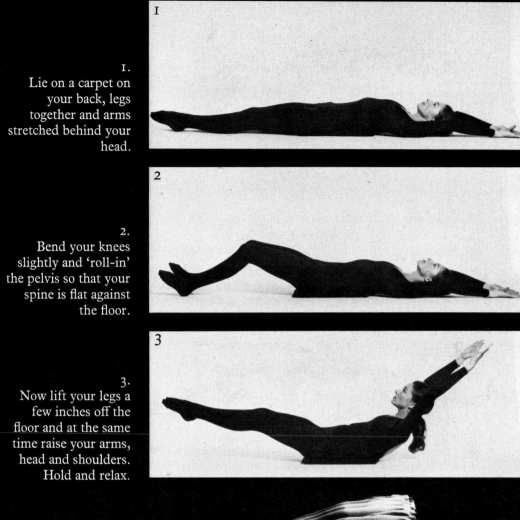

I

1.
Lie on a carpet on your back, legs together and arms stretched behind your head.

2

2.
Bend your knees slightly and 'roll-in' the pelvis so that your spine is flat against the floor.

3

3.
Now lift your legs a few inches off the floor and at the same time raise your arms, head and shoulders. Hold and relax.

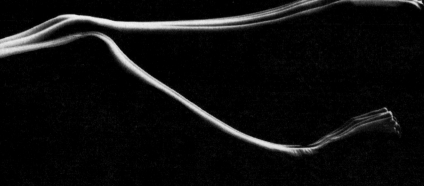

It is most important that the small of your back remains *hard* against the floor when you lift your legs and arms. If your spine curves away from the floor as you stretch up – stop immediately. This is dangerous, because your stomach has stopped exercising and your lower back is taking the strain.

Stomach and Thighs

The exercises in this section are primarily designed to shape
and firm the thighs, but they also help to strengthen and
tighten the muscles of the stomach. These exercises are very
hard and will undoubtedly produce groans of agony! But do
not use this as an excuse to skip them, because they really do
produce fantastic results.

One pupil who has found that it pays to persevere is
actress Toby Robins, who has regained her figure after three
children. She agrees that 'Lotte's exercises are extremely
tough, sometimes they are painful and you don't want to do
them, but they are marvellous for the figure and do you so
much good.'

So practise and master these exercises, then have fun by
working out your own routine, flowing from one exercise
into another. Just remember that if you stop between these
exercises, always start again with your knees bent (see
position 1, exercise 22) and then you will never strain your
back.

Exercise 19

1.
Sit on a carpet with your lower back against a wall. Open your legs, bend your knees and place fingertips on the floor in front of you.

2–4.
Lean on your hands, raise both legs, then straighten and str-e-tch your legs and really point those toes! Relax and repeat three times, gradually increasing to eight.

As you get stronger, try to repeat movements 2 and 3 five times, while keeping your legs in the air.

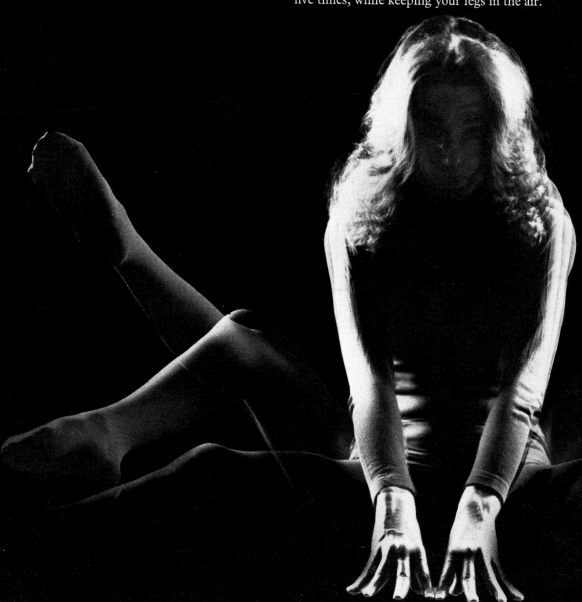

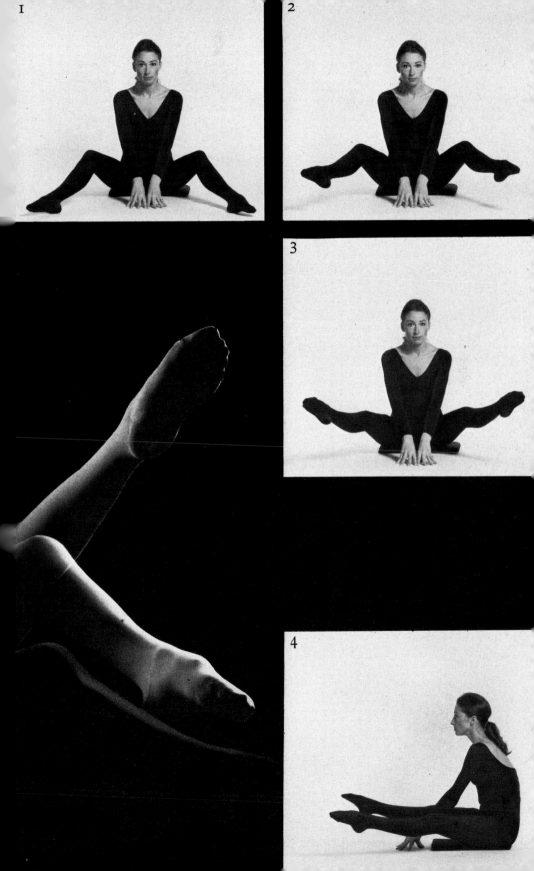

Exercise 20

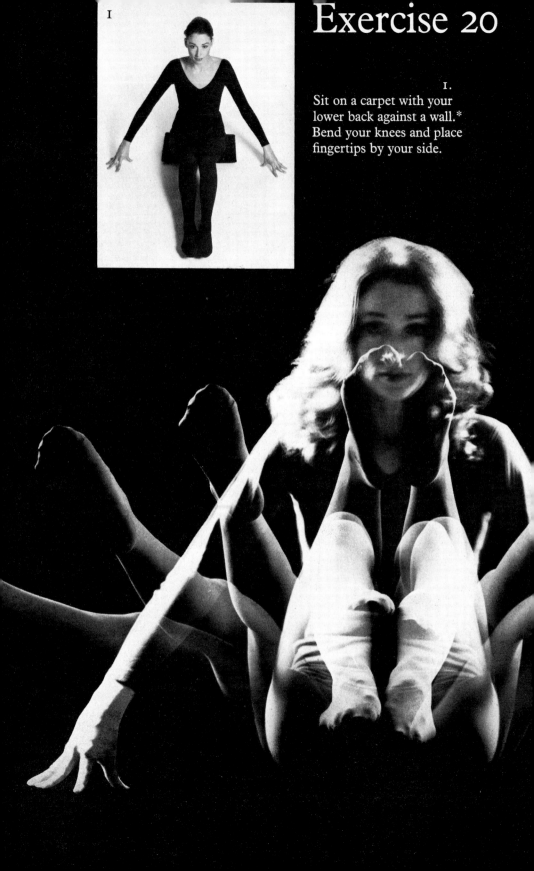

I.

Sit on a carpet with your lower back against a wall.* Bend your knees and place fingertips by your side.

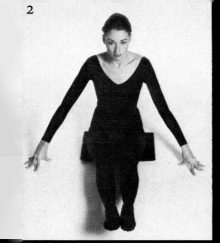 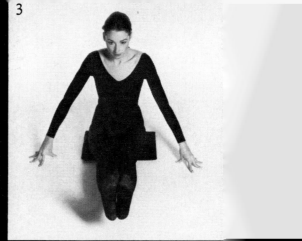

2.

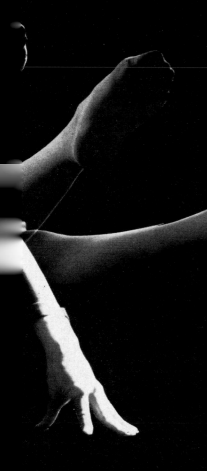

Press the small of your back into the w
lean on your hands and raise both legs
off the floor. Some people will only be
able to raise their legs a few inches,
others will be able to come up higher.

3.
Straighten your legs and pull feet hard
towards you.

4.
Now keeping your legs straight, open
and close your legs as wide as possible.
Try and start with three open/close
movements and build up to twenty.

*If your stomach muscles are not stron
you may have to start by leaning agains
and bringing your lower back slightly a
the wall. Only adopt this position while
strengthen your stomach, and go back t
sitting position, above, as soon as you c

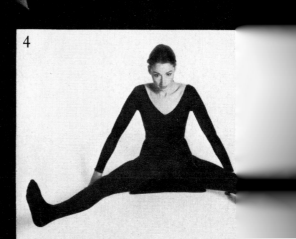

Exercise 21

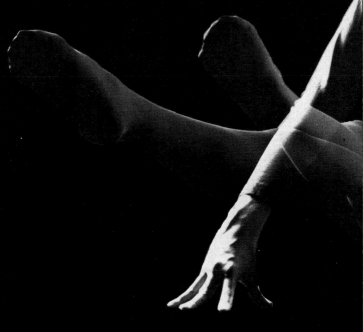

1.
Sit as for exercise 20.

2.
Lean on your hands and raise both legs a few inches off the floor.

3 & 4.
Now straighten legs, point toes hard, and make small scissor movements with your legs, crossing at the ankles. Try and start with three/five small scissor movements, and gradually increase to twenty.

5.
As you get stronger you can progress to a wide scissor movement, again starting at five and building up to twenty.

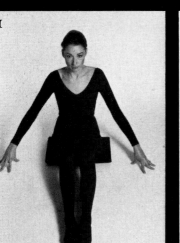

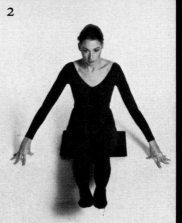

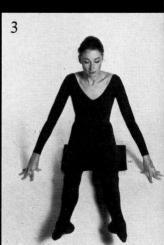

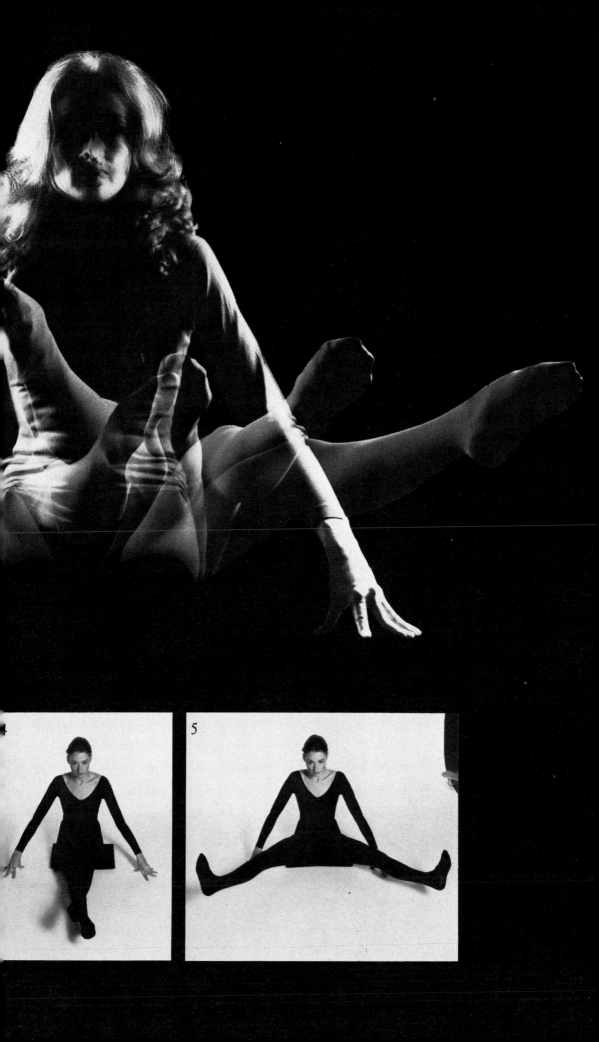

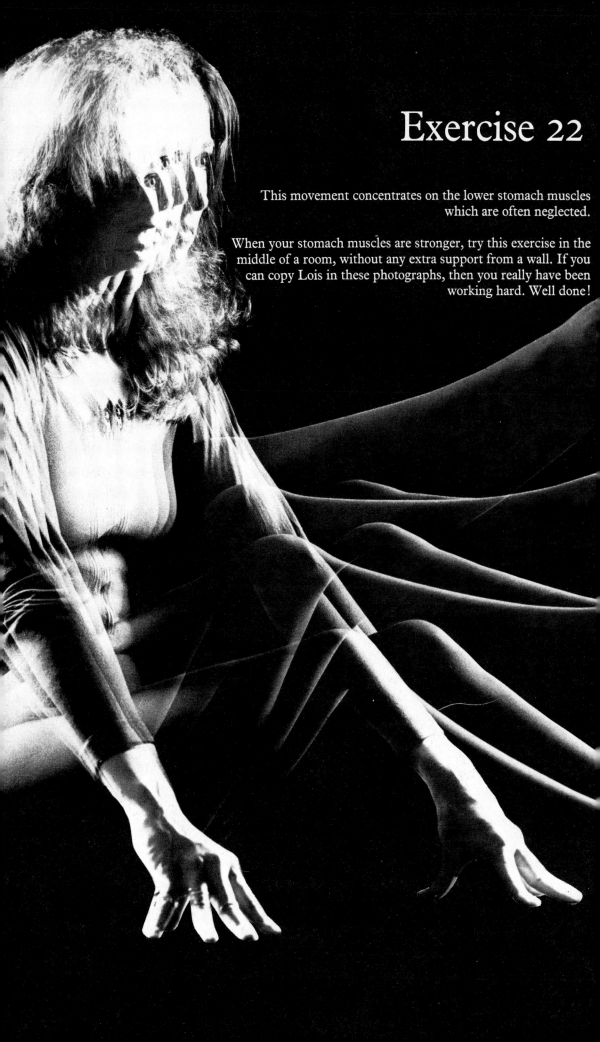

Exercise 22

This movement concentrates on the lower stomach muscles which are often neglected.

When your stomach muscles are stronger, try this exercise in the middle of a room, without any extra support from a wall. If you can copy Lois in these photographs, then you really have been working hard. Well done!

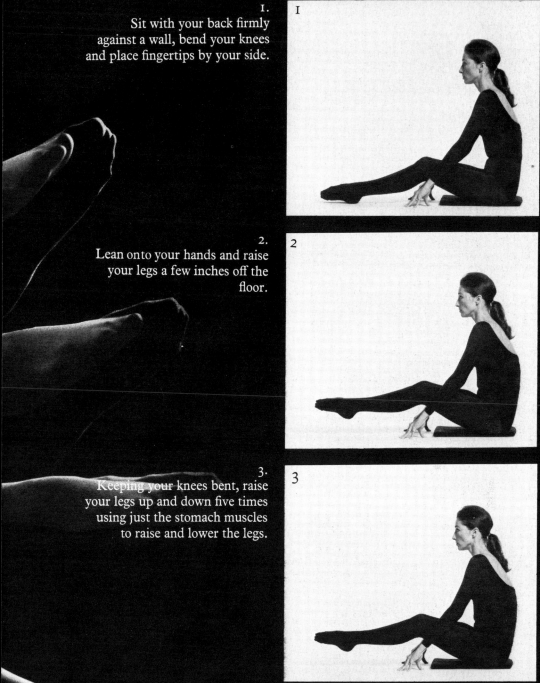

1.
Sit with your back firmly against a wall, bend your knees and place fingertips by your side.

2.
Lean onto your hands and raise your legs a few inches off the floor.

3.
Keeping your knees bent, raise your legs up and down five times using just the stomach muscles to raise and lower the legs.

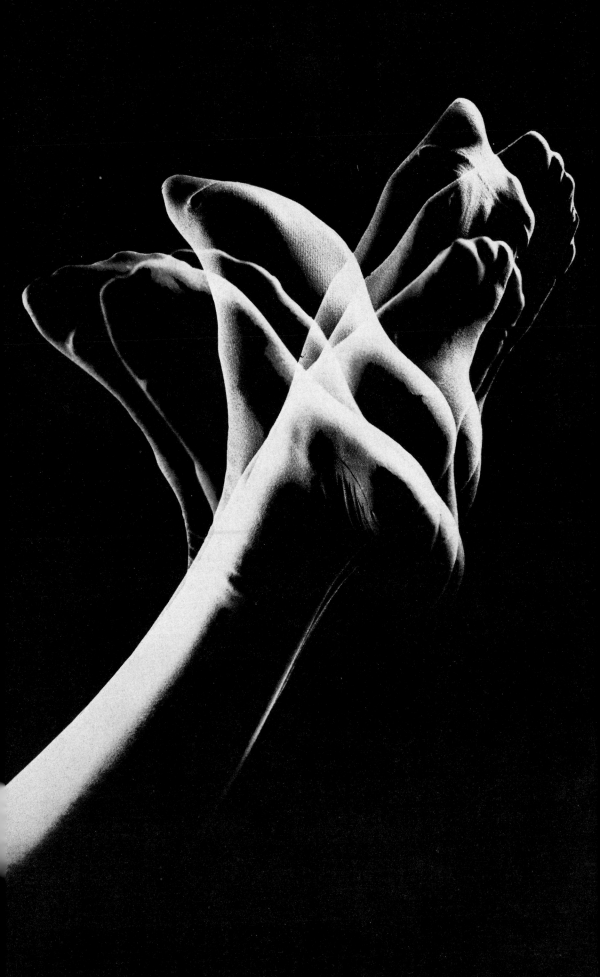

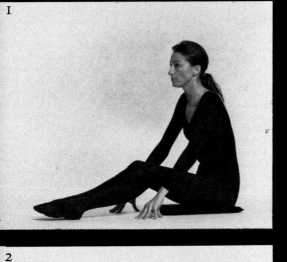

1.
Sit as in exercise 20.

2.
Lean onto your hands,
raise both legs off
the floor, then
straighten legs and
point your toes.

3.
Now circle both feet
together, clockwise (ten times),
then anti-clockwise (ten times).

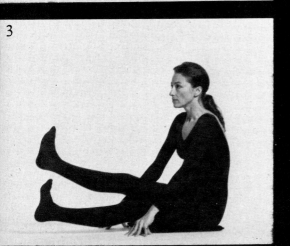

Bottoms

Women who sit all day can easily suffer from a
'hanging-bottom', but a soft, flabby bottom can easily be
tightened into a firm sexy 'derrière' if you concentrate on the
exercises in this section. The cheeks of your bottom will
tighten and 'lift' and the two pads of fat that tend to sit
below the waist (on your rear side) will flatten and smooth
away.

Some of the exercises in this section are done whilst
holding on to the back of a chair for support, and you should
always make sure that your chair is pushed firmly against a
wall, so that it doesn't topple or slide away from you.

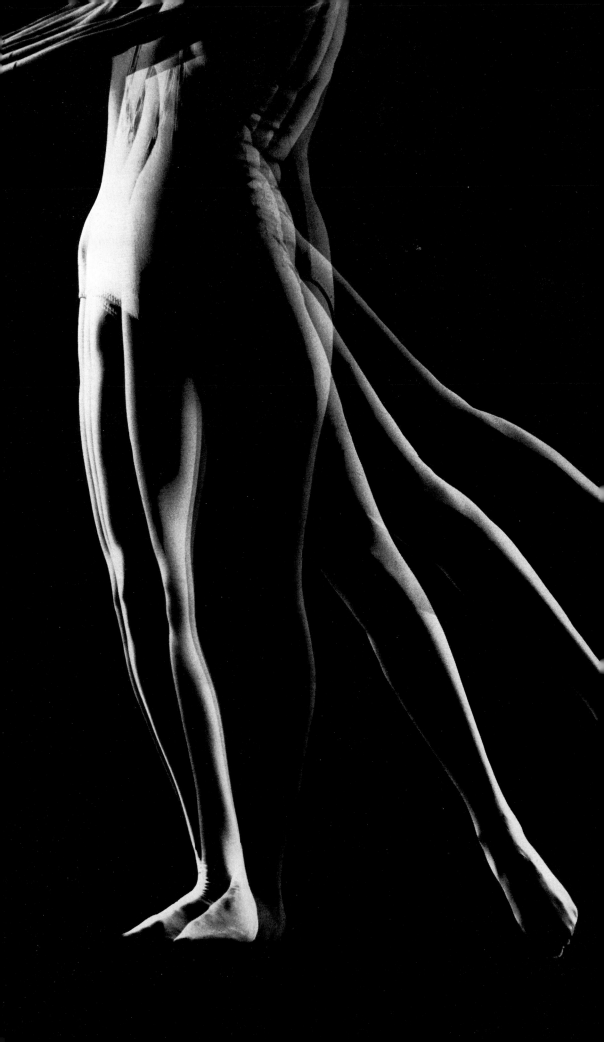

Exercise 24

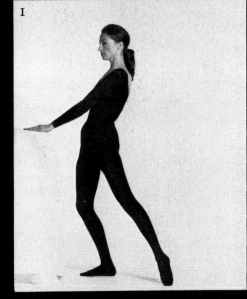

1.
Hold on to the back of a chair, tuck your bottom under and push the pelvic bone forward against the chair. Extend your left leg to the side, bend both legs slightly and lean over the extended leg.

2 & 3.
Keeping the pelvis pushed forward and both legs slightly bent, now roll the left hip into the chair, then raise and lower the left leg, five times – and keep leaning over that leg! Repeat the other side.

Do not cheat by moving just the lower leg from the knee joint – remember that the whole leg is raised and lowered from the hip.

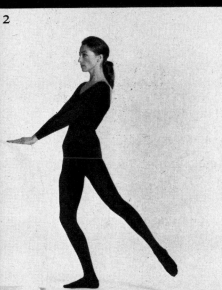

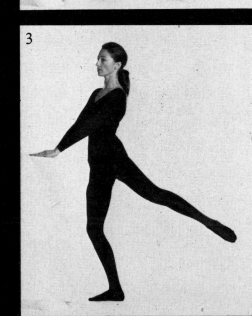

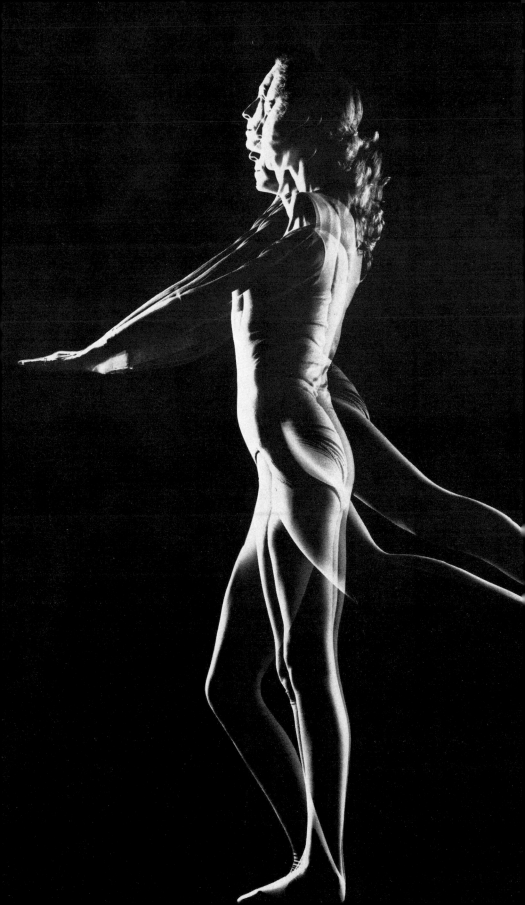

Exercise 25

1.
Hold on to the back of a chair, bend both legs and lean into your right leg. Keeping the left leg bent, push it behind you, point the toes, lift your left leg as high as possible and lean slightly over the raised leg.

2.
Now straighten both legs hard.

3.
Keep leaning slightly over the left leg, now bend both legs again but do not drop the left leg – keep it as high as possible.

Repeat positions 2 and 3 five times, then repeat with the right leg raised.

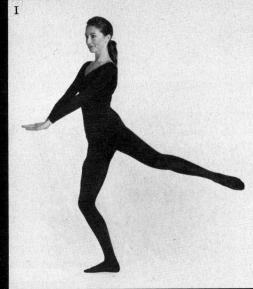

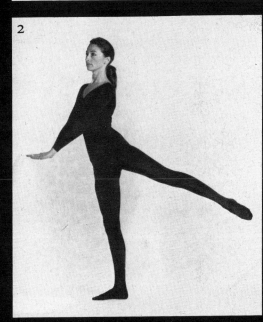

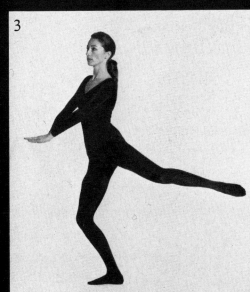

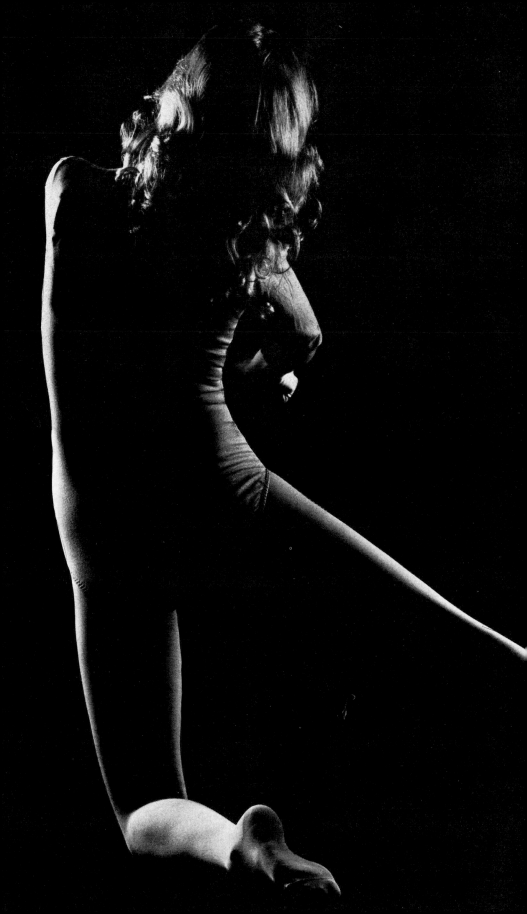

Exercise 26

1.
Kneel on a carpet and hold on to the edge of a table. Kneeling on the right knee, extend your left leg diagonally behind you with the knee slightly bent and lean over the extended leg.

2.
Without moving the body – do not lean away from the extended leg – now roll the left hip forwards, then raise and lower the whole leg off the floor five times.

This is a hip movement and if you are doing the exercise correctly, you will only be able to raise the leg a few inches. Repeat with the other leg.

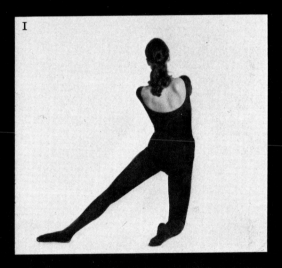

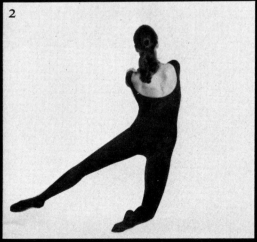

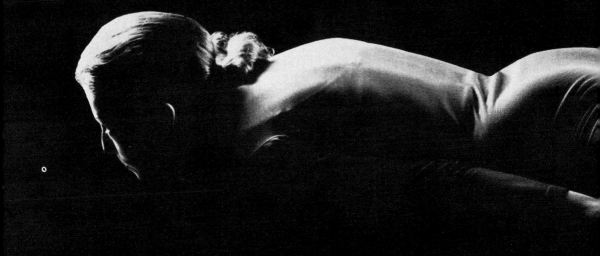

Exercise 27

It is important to keep
your chin on the carpet
throughout this exercise,
to ensure that there is no
strain on your back.

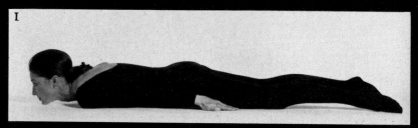

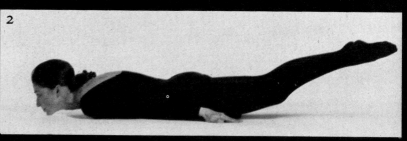

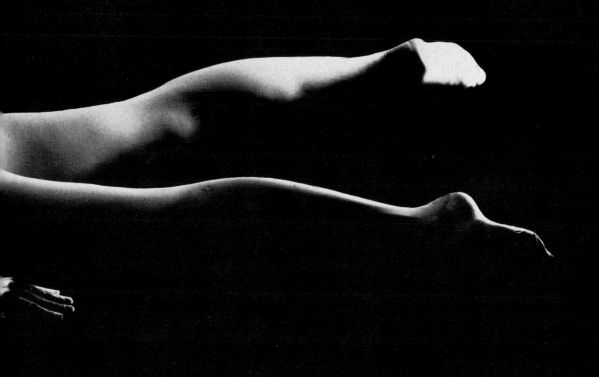

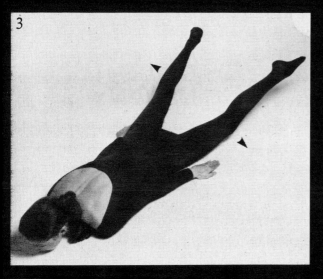

1.
Lie on a carpet on your
stomach, and rest your chin
on the floor. Place your
hands by your side with
palms face down.

2.
Open legs wide and raise
both legs off the floor, with
knees slightly bent.

3.
Now with little pushes
from the thighs, open your
legs wider. Push open,
open, open, open. Relax
and repeat twice more.

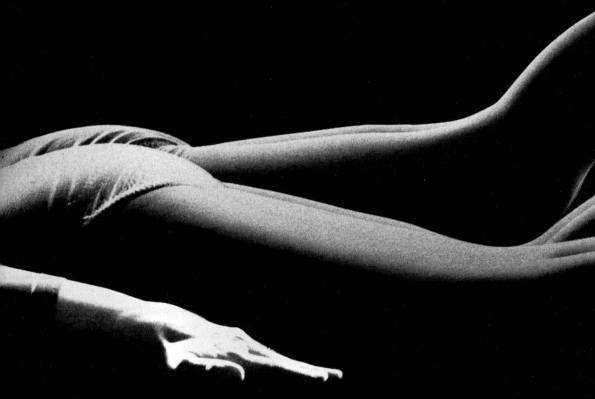

Exercise 28

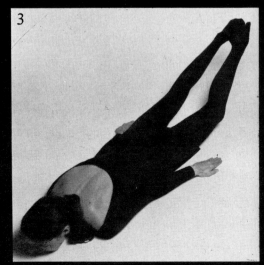

3

Lie on a carpet as for exercise 27,
and remember to keep your chin
firmly on the floor.

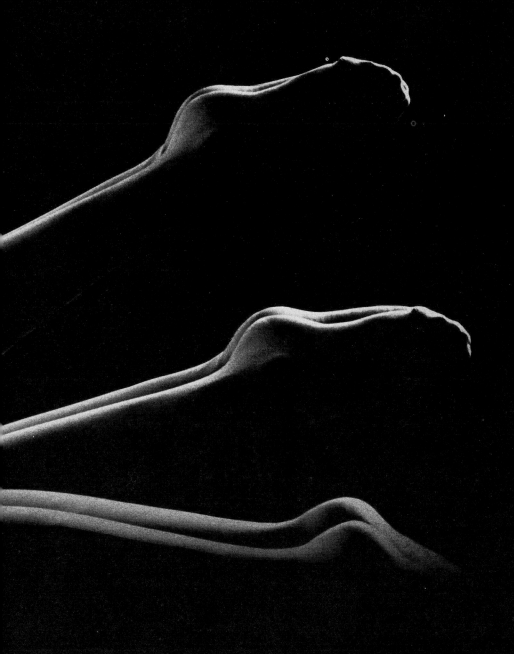

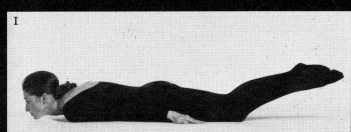

1

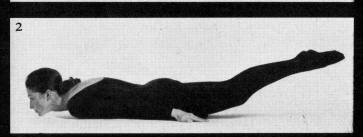

2

1 & 2.
Bring the soles
of your feet
together.

3.
Now keeping your
feet together,
raise your legs
up and down
eight times.
Relax and repeat
twice more.

Stretching

Stretching makes your body loose and graceful and gives you a feeling of vitality that shows in the way you walk.

With inactivity, your muscles will contract as you grow older – you will stoop, develop stiffness, aches and pains. But all this can be avoided and you can allay the fear of growing old by keeping your muscles stretched, strong and supple.

Lotte Berk is a perfect example of how exercise keeps the body youthful and agile. So stretch every day – but remember to warm-up first and include those important neck stretching exercises in your warm-up routine.

Exercise 29

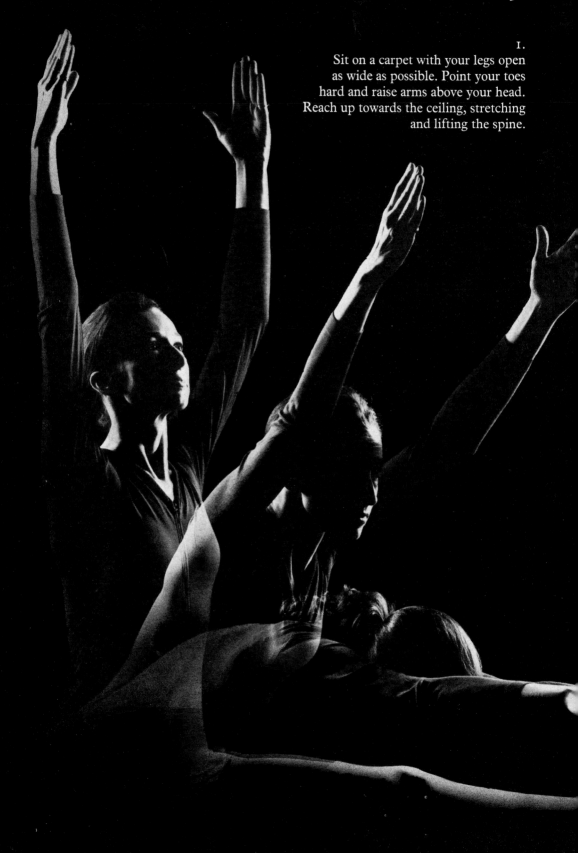

1.

Sit on a carpet with your legs open as wide as possible. Point your toes hard and raise arms above your head. Reach up towards the ceiling, stretching and lifting the spine.

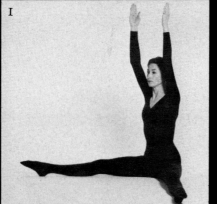

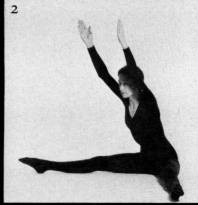

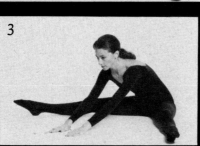

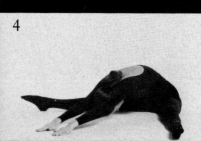

2.
Now bend forward from the hips, keeping your back straight. This is a hip movement – so do not lean forwards merely by rounding the spine!

3 & 4.
Stretch forwards as far as possible and place your palms on the floor between your legs. Gently slide your palms further away – go as far as possible – really str-e-tch and hold this position to the count of five. Can you feel your inner thigh muscles being stretched? Good!

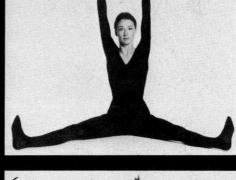

5.
As your hip-joints get looser you can vary the exercise by sitting tall and pulling the feet towards you.

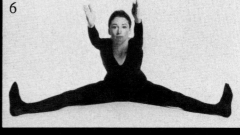

6 & 7.
Now stretch forward, keeping the feet pulled towards you, bend down to reach for your feet and touch the floor with your head.

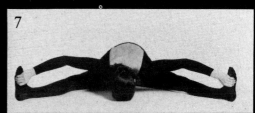

Exercise 30

1.
Sit on a carpet on the floor. Stretch up to the ceiling, pull your feet towards you and press your knee-caps hard into the carpet, so that your feet pop off the floor.

2.
Now turn to face your left foot and stretch out.

3.
Lean over to take hold of your foot, try to get your head as low as possible and if you are supple you should get your head down to your knee. Sit up again and repeat the other side.

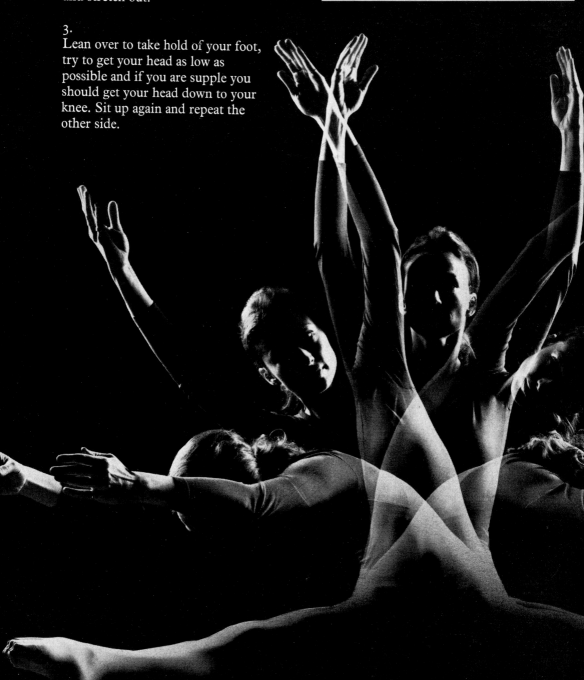

2

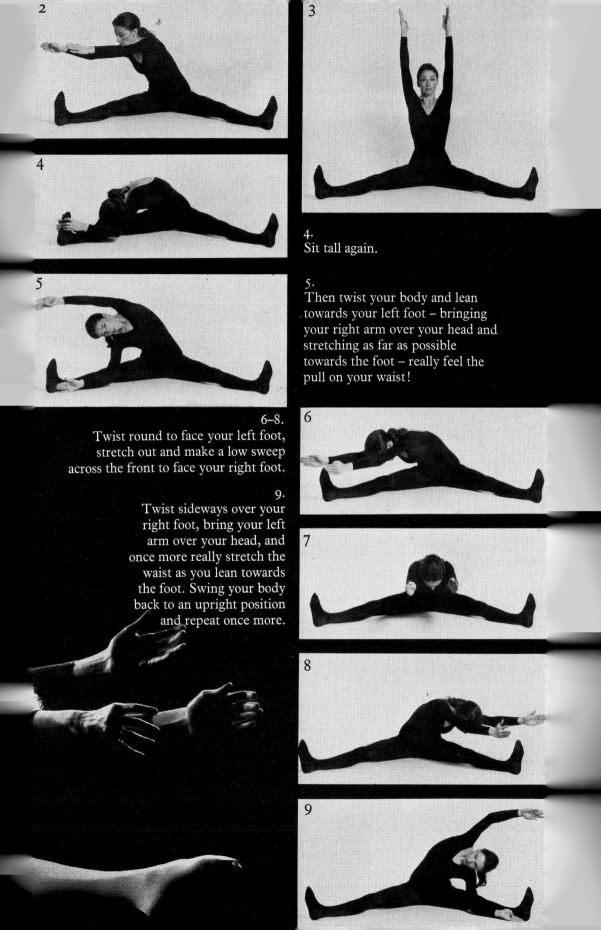

3

4.
Sit tall again.

4

5.
Then twist your body and lean towards your left foot – bringing your right arm over your head and stretching as far as possible towards the foot – really feel the pull on your waist!

5

6–8.
Twist round to face your left foot, stretch out and make a low sweep across the front to face your right foot.

6

9.
Twist sideways over your right foot, bring your left arm over your head, and once more really stretch the waist as you lean towards the foot. Swing your body back to an upright position and repeat once more.

7

8

9

Exercise 31

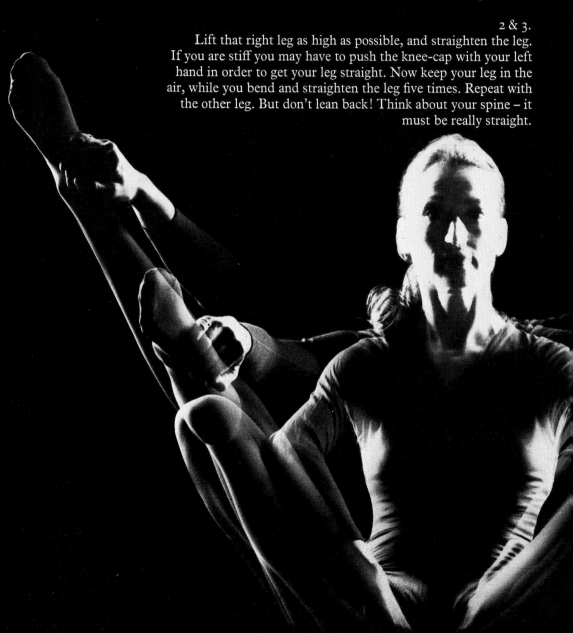

1.

Sit on a carpet with your legs extended in front of you. Keep your back really straight and take hold of your right instep with your right hand.

2 & 3.

Lift that right leg as high as possible, and straighten the leg. If you are stiff you may have to push the knee-cap with your left hand in order to get your leg straight. Now keep your leg in the air, while you bend and straighten the leg five times. Repeat with the other leg. But don't lean back! Think about your spine – it must be really straight.

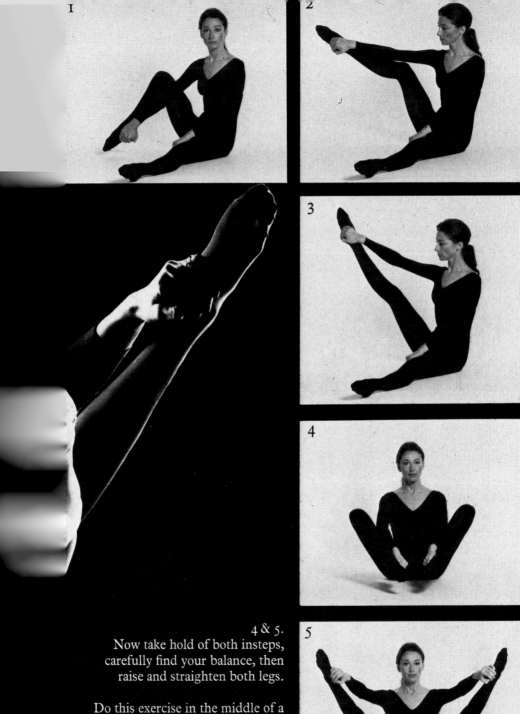

4 & 5.
Now take hold of both insteps,
carefully find your balance, then
raise and straighten both legs.

Do this exercise in the middle of a
room, in case you fall backwards.
As you get fitter, and gain control
of your balance, you will be able to
raise and straighten both legs,
whilst keeping your back upright
and perfectly still

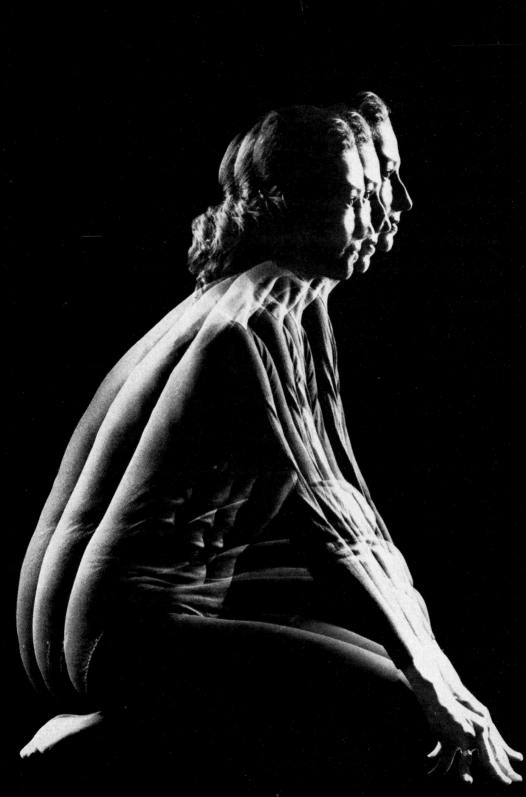

Exercise 32

The muscles on your instep can easily shorten and contract with age and inactivity. Old people who suffer this way are forced to 'shuffle' along instead of walking smoothly. So we call this exercis 'old woman's walk' – but it is in fact, how to avoid old woman's walk.

1.
Sit on your feet, lean slightly forwards and rest on your fingertips.

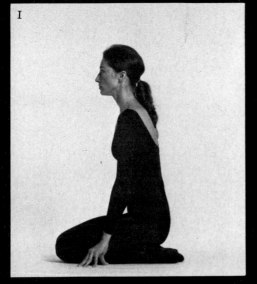

2.
Now lean onto your hands and raise your knees off the ground. Hold this position to a count of three, and lower. Repeat five/ten times.

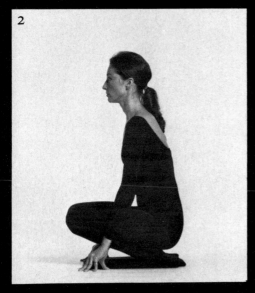

3.
As your feet get supple, you wil be able to raise the knees higher like this.

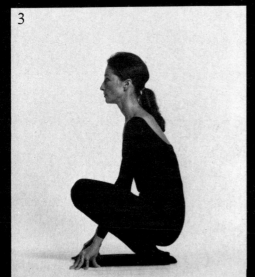

Spinal Stretch

To cure a back ache you must exercise it. A bad back is the greatest excuse for lying down and resting, but this is so wrong. Get up – exercise, and you will discover that correct exercise movements can remove the pain without the need for pain-killers.

The following spinal stretching movements are based on orthopaedic exercises. They are perfectly safe to do and there is absolutely no way you can hurt your back. They have been specially devised to gently manipulate and move the spine so that aches and pains can be cured naturally.

If you are still in doubt, go back to the chapter 'Why Exercise is so Important' and read the words of Dr Guy Beauchamp which confirm that strains in the mid or lower back region *can* be relieved with regular exercise.

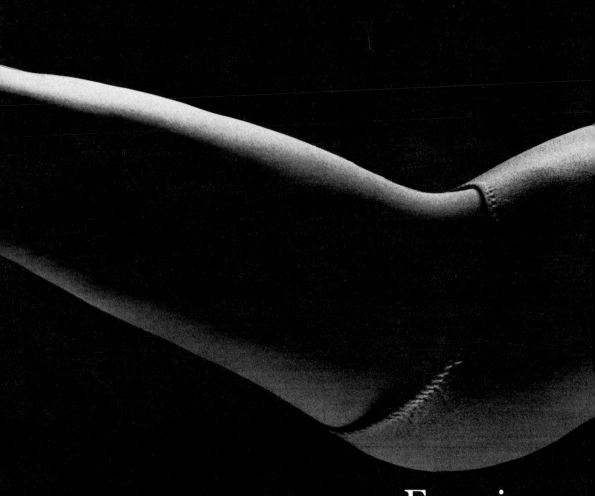

Exercise 33

This simple spinal stretch can be done at home to ease an
aching back, in your hotel room to unwind after a hectic
day – or after a walk through Paris, over all those
'cobble' stones!

1.
Lie on a carpet on your back, stretch arms above your
head and bend your knees.

2.
Now 'roll-in' the pelvis and push your spine hard against
the floor, so that your bottom comes slightly off the floor.
Hold this position for a count of three, relax and repeat.

Continue repeating this exercise until the ache and
stiffness in your back begins to ease.

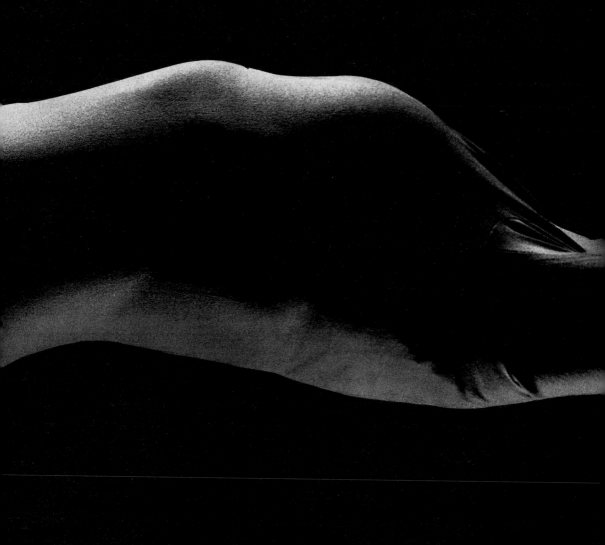

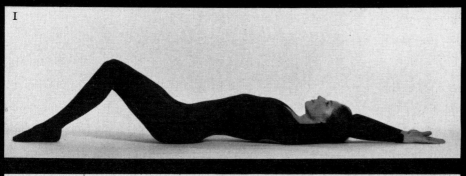

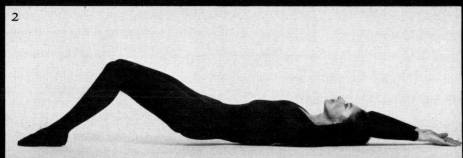

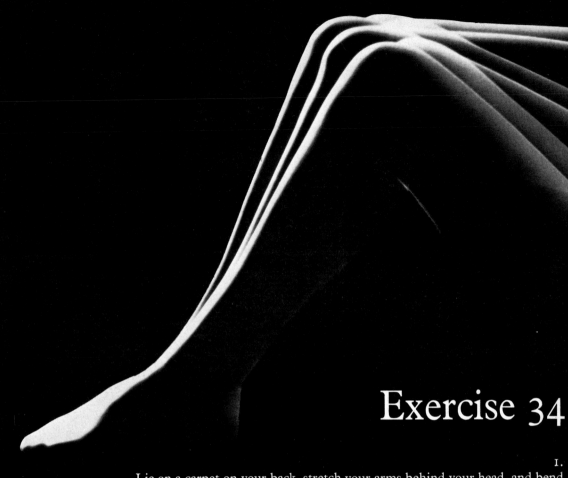

Exercise 34

I.
Lie on a carpet on your back, stretch your arms behind your head, and bend the knees.

2.
Now keep your feet flat on the floor, lift your bottom and push the pelvic bone up as high as possible. Your arms, head, shoulders – and feet – remain on the floor.

3.
As you *slowly* lower your body, stretch the spine as if you were pushing your bottom towards your feet.

4.
Now 'roll-in' your pelvis, pushing your spine hard against the floor so that your bottom comes an inch off the floor.

Relax and repeat.

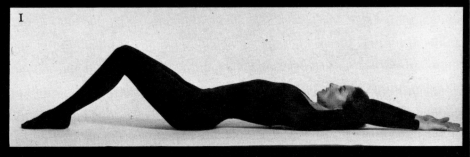

I

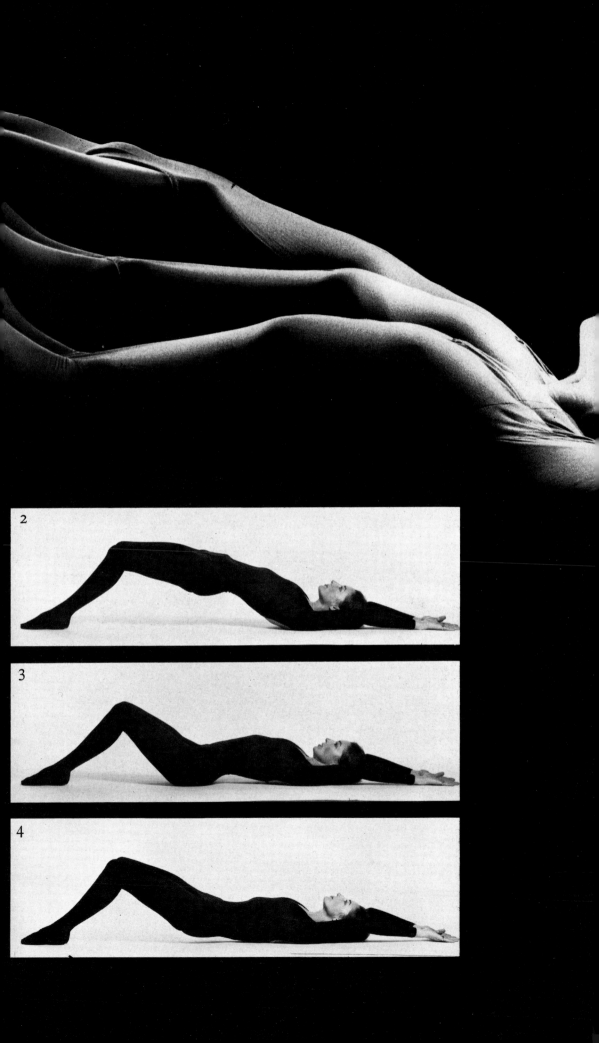